Emerging You

A New Path to Leaving the Past Behind, Finding Your Purpose, and Becoming the Best Version of You

By

Soodabeh Mokry, RN, CHt

Editing: Amber Torres
Cover Design: Defining Moments Press, Inc
Author's Photo Courtesy Of: Kate Singh Photography

Dedication

I dedicate this book to my grandparents, my father, and my brother, who are my guardian angels in the spirit world.

Acknowledgements

To my mother, who loved me unconditionally and tried her best to make sure her children had a wonderful life.

To my amazing son and daughter who have always loved me unconditionally and supported me throughout my life journey. I live and breathe because of you two.

To my daughter-in-law and my amazing granddaughters who bring me love and joy every day. I love you, I am proud of you, and I am a better person because of you.

To my brothers, sister- in- laws, niece, nephews, and all of my family in Iran who accepted me just the way I am. I love you so much, and I am proud of each and every one of you.

To my teachers, coaches, and mentors who helped me to discover and embrace the new and best version of me.

To my editor, Kristin Thiel, who has been a crucial part of my journey for the past 4 years. Thank you for your loving nature, wisdom, and guidance.

To the Defining Moments team of experts, Melanie Warner and the fabulous Amber Torres. Thank you for your love and support.

And to my clients, patients, and their families who accepted me by opening their homes, their hearts, and allowing me to serve. It is through our many interactions that I have learned to be a better mentor.

Contents

Introduction

It doesn't matter where you grew up, who your parents are, where you went to school, or what others think of you. What matters the most is that you recognize your self-worth and believe in yourself. Remember who you really are: a powerful spirit in human form. You are resilient, you are brilliant, you are significant. You are in control and able to make wise decisions. You can even use your obstacles as stepping stones to get to where you need to be in life. The power to choose what is best for *you* is what allows you to create the life you want and truly deserve.

You are not a victim, you are not broken, and you are not destined to suffer. Life is not a fairytale and it is not always easy; it can be challenging with ebbs and flows. However, the struggles are temporary. You may feel powerless when losing a loved one, dealing with health issues, or mourning for a relationship or job that has ended. However, in the midst of these challenges, you always have the following choice: to move forward with forgiveness, healing, and love to lead the life you desire or to harbor guilt and shame, leading to a life filled with regret, anger, and resentment.

Feeling restless or discontented regarding your circumstances is a direct indication that things need to change. These emotions warn you that you have detoured from where you need to be in life. It means that you are not in alignment with your spirit and what brings you joy and happiness. You have forgotten the powerful spirit that resides within you. You have forgotten the guidance of your intuition; the infinite wisdom bestowed upon you by the Divine Source-the Creator.

Your current life is a direct result of the choices you have made. It's based on the challenges you have faced and the triumphs you experienced. You have created this life thus far. It's not about blame, shame, or feeling guilty. It's about accountability and taking responsibility for your actions. Your current lifestyle and what you choose to do every day determines your future. So, if you are not satisfied with your current situation and wish for something different, you need to begin changing the way you think, act, and react every day.

Do you believe you are the victim of a series of unfortunate events? Do you blame your parents, family, friends, partners, or society for your lack of success? Do you believe you were born to suffer?

As long as you have the victim mentality, you will always attract experiences that prove you are a victim. Living with the victim mindset diminishes your power. Your negative thoughts and beliefs about yourself, attract more of the same sort of experiences. The thoughts of "not good enough," "not worthy enough," "not young enough," "not tall enough," are only preventing you from experiencing the life you are meant to live.

You are not destined to be alone, poor, or powerless. You are not destined to be the victim of a chain of unfortunate events. You are responsible for your current life, and you own the power to change it. You have the capacity to choose a better life; to believe that there are better ways to live. It's time to raise your standard and take steps to enhance the quality of your life. It's about mastering the journey of self-love. This journey starts with believing you are worthy of having a better future. This journey starts with believing you are victorious.

The possibilities are endless when you decide to change. The power to change is in your capable hands. The divine light, love, and wisdom are within you; they are your birthright. The power was bestowed upon you from the moment you were created. You are capable of choosing what you want. You have the freedom to take the steps toward creating the best life and achieving your goals, dreams, and heart's desires. The action steps you take today will pave the way to a brighter future.

It's time to start loving and believing in yourself. This book is about the journey of self-love. The path to lead with a heart filled with love, compassion, and peace. Loving yourself is not about being selfish or self-centered. Instead, it is a powerful extension of the infinite love originating from the Divine Source. Loving yourself allows you to love and accept others.

Choose you. Love you. That ultimate choice will take you where you need to be; on the path to discover the new version of you. In this book, *Emerging You*, I will teach you how to become happy, healthy, and fulfilled in all aspects of life.

It's time to create your destiny...

Chapter One
The Crossroads

I stood at the crossroads. When I first arrived in the United States, It was the darkest time of my life. I was faced with the most challenging experiences I had ever had to endure. I had waited three years to be reunited with Hameed, my husband of ten years. We had two children together. I had sacrificed my safety, my job, and my family to join him in our new home in the US from our old home in Iran. Now, it felt like I had wasted, rather than given, so much time, energy, and money to be here, to be happy, to be free.

I was living with a man whom I no longer knew and, perhaps even worse, who no longer seemed to recognize me. I had to take a step – but which way?

A Stranger in My Home

For two weeks in my new home, I could not have told you what was wrong- I just knew that something was very, very wrong. I had expected a thrilled and relieved greeting at the airport. Instead, the children and I arrived to find Hameed circling the pickup zone outside the terminal, and even then, though he embraced them, he barely touched me. There was little conversation, barely any contact. I remember the *thunk-swish-thunk* of the windshield wipers in the long stretches of silence during our car ride home. As I laid in bed that night, the inches between Hameed's body and mine felt greater than the thousands of miles we had been experiencing. I told myself that this was strange for all of us and that tomorrow would be better.

As the days passed, I learned quickly that tomorrow would never be better. Unable to sleep, I'd get up early each morning and sit on a chair in the kitchen, looking outside. I had barely memorized my new address, barely knew exactly where I was, let alone where I was in the bigger picture of life. I had no idea how to navigate the streets to grocery stores, a doctor, the children's school. It continued to rain, making me more depressed. At first, I felt as if the whole world were crying for the pain I carried in my heart and soul. Gradually, grief and anxiety turned into anger; I was sick and tired of walking on eggshells trying to make Hameed happy. I had been doing that for years.

Sitting on the old chair in the old kitchen in my new home, I yearned for Hameed to appear in the doorway. To come to me and hold me in his arms, kiss me, and tell me that he loved me, that he couldn't live without me. I desired to hear the words he used to write in his love letters, promising a beautiful future. I wanted my life back.

The silence in the home and the sound of the rain created a hypnotic state, taking me back to a dark time I had experienced twelve years prior, one year after the revolution took place in Iran. Hameed and I had been dating for a year then. My mother was against us *dating*. It wasn't culturally acceptable; in Iran, one was either single or married-not intentionally remaining in the interim. She also believed we were too young. I was nineteen years old, and Hameed was eighteen. I was supposed to marry someone my mother had chosen for me rather than dating and marrying the one I loved.

And first, I was supposed to have earned a degree. My mother wanted me to go to college, receive a higher education, and be independent to provide for myself. She was a teacher and firm about raising educated children. Life had taught my mother a valuable lesson when we lost my father years before when I was thirteen years old. My mother had to work two jobs to provide for us.

During this time, she came to understand quite clearly that you cannot count on a man to provide for you. Women must maintain the ability to be financially independent- even if they are married.

"You never know what challenges you will face in life," Mother said after I told her about Hameed. "What would we have done if I weren't a teacher and was unable to work after your father died? You need to go to college first, and find a good job, and then the right man will find you."

Mother managed to convince me to attend a nursing school across the country. It was heartbreaking for me to move away from Hameed, but he promised that us staying together over the distance would prove to my mother that he really loved me. "Don't worry, Soodabeh – we can make it. I want your mother to know that I want the best for you too," Hameed said.

During my first term at nursing school, we heard the government was planning to close all the universities and colleges in the country. Students and teachers who did not believe in the government's religious ideology would not be allowed back in when schools reopened – if they reopened. It seemed as though Iran were moving backward, even that it might entirely reject its history as one of the most educated countries on the planet. But it wouldn't close our schools indefinitely without a fight from us. A nationwide protest was scheduled: on the same day, all students, and teachers, all over Iran would protest. Hameed had persuaded me to join the movement.

"I will join the protest here right after taking my midterm exam," I told Hameed the day before the protest.

The next day, I lounged on the stairs of the university's front entrance, talking with my friends. We were still teenagers – it felt like nothing to our youthful systems to socialize, take a test, and protest, all in one day. Suddenly, we heard gunshots; one after another, followed by screaming. Everyone was terrified, running to find a safe place to hide, not knowing what had happened. My friends and I found ourselves in the courtyard, but we were not safe there. We were quickly mobbed, surrounded by violent, angry men and women with guns, baseball bats, knives, and rocks. They hit us on the heads, arms, legs, everywhere.

Then, I felt a strong hand push me from the back, and I fell onto the cement. They continued beating me. I gasped for air as others fell on top of me. Then the weight started to be lifted; the people on top of me were being dragged away. I heard their screams for their captors to release them. And then I was lifted roughly from the ground. They threw us in a truck, pointing their big guns at us, screaming profanities. I was frightened, thinking about my mom, who had no idea where I was. *What will she do if I die? And Hameed-what is happening to him?* I thought.

It was a hot summer day; we were all soaked with sweat and getting hotter by the second because we were crammed together with no room to move at all. Everyone was quiet, afraid to say anything. I could feel my heart beating alarmingly fast in my chest. My head was pounding and throbbing from the pain. I couldn't stop thinking about air and how there seemed to be none. There was no space between us; it seemed as if we were one big pile of flesh.

The truck stopped, and I heard the sound of a large metal door opening. When the truck's door flew open, all we could see were guns pointed at us, and there was shouting for us to get out of the truck. We entered a yard that was more than ten feet long and surrounded by tall, dark brown and red brick walls. There were several male guards, dressed in green army uniforms, with short, dark hair and thick black beards, their faces red and eyes bulging. They were shouting, "Go, go, go! Move, move!" They led us into a dark room about the size of a basketball court. There was one small window, with vertical black metal bars, very high near the ceiling. We couldn't see anything outside the window, and no one outside could see what was going on inside that room.

Without air-conditioning or a fan, the room quickly filled with the foul odor of sweat mixed with vomit and urine. I wanted to throw up. One of the guards shoved me and I fell. I got up and tucked myself into a far corner. I looked around the room, at the many other bloodied or bowed faces. I was filled with terror; my body shook uncontrollably, and tears streamed down my face.

My head felt like it was about to explode as the sharp pain at the back of my skull grew. I started hyperventilating. Shortly after, I felt the room spinning, and my eyes blurred. I could hear ringing in my ears as I slumped to the floor unconscious.

And I Survived

I felt a sharp pain in my nostrils and, all of a sudden, felt the liquid – blood- running down my face. I opened my eyes and saw a man right in front of my face. I tried to lift my hands or move my body to stop him, but I couldn't; I was very weak. I choked on my sobs because whatever he was doing was clogging my nose. He stopped what he was doing and stared at me.

"Oh, she is alive," he whispered and walked out of the room. As he moved away, I saw he was wearing a white doctor's coat.

I carefully moved my fingers to feel about my face – I guessed he had stuck oxygen tubes in my nose.

I was lying in a bed with metal side rails in a white room without windows or pictures. I was covered with white sheets and a brown woolen blanket. There was a dull metal pole to the left side of the bed, an intravenous fluid bag hanging from it with its clear plastic tube running all the way to a vein inside my left arm. There was a large green oxygen tank on the right side of the bed attached to the white plastic tubing that was in my nostrils.

I was scared. I didn't know what had happened or how I had gotten to the hospital, not even what hospital I was in. I wept quietly.

I had been raised Muslim and grew up with a strong faith in God. I was taught that God was love, light, merciful, and kind. I believed that he would answer our prayers, protect us, support us, provide for us, and keep us safe from harm. So, how could it be possible that the new regime was terrorizing and killing people, including innocent young students, in the name of God and Islam? I could not comprehend how cruel they could be, using religious beliefs to get what they wanted.

I don't know how long I lay there with no one looking in on me – it must have been hours –but then the door opened, and my heart soared. My mom and my cousin ran in with tears in their eyes. I had no idea how they had found me, but I was so glad to see them.

"Mom! Is that you? How did you get here? Where am I?"

"Oh, thank God you are alive. We have been searching everywhere for you," said my mom. "You have been in a coma for the past week. We don't know what exactly happened or how you got here."

Together, we learned that I had been in a coma due to a severe head injury. Still, there was a security guard right outside of my hospital room, planning to take me back to jail as soon as I was well enough to be transported.

My cousin and her husband were well-known in the medical community in Ahvaz. They were able to convince the authorities that I had been at the protest to help injured people, since I was a nursing student. With the grace of God, I was able to get discharged and go to my cousin's home that day and back to Tehran with my mom a few days later. I had no idea what happened to any of my friends or classmates.

I had nightmares every night. I would wake up soaked in sweat from the terror of remembering the gun-shots, the blood, the crying, and the sounds of people screaming in torture. I was afraid of going anywhere without my mom, and every little noise made me jump. I was paralyzed by fear and unable to move forward; I couldn't even take care of myself without help.

"Mom, can you sit here while I am taking a shower? I am scared. Please don't close the door, Mom," I would cry in fear.

"I am here, honey. No one could ever hurt you, I promise," she would respond.

My mom was getting exhausted and angry, blaming Hameed for everything that had happened to me. "I raised you right, and kept you safe. I taught you how to behave and what to do so you wouldn't be in this situation. Do you have any idea what you have done to me? Can you even imagine how I felt, not knowing if you were dead or alive, or where you were for an entire week? Are you going to stop seeing that stupid boy now?"

My family told me that I was lucky to have survived. "They raped and killed many students. They cut their bodies and threw them in the river to die. It's just a miracle that you weren't one of them. We don't know what you were thinking!"

I was paranoid, but I did not regret going to the protest. "I only wanted democracy, freedom of choice and speech, to go to school and have a better life. I wanted to be with my friends and other students to show support, and to prove that we need freedom and education. We didn't deserve to be treated that way. I didn't deserve to be tortured that way – no one did," I declared.

How I Came to Live in the United States

I remembered the night Hameed told me he had to flee Iran three years ago. We had just finished eating dinner. Our Son, Cyrus, had run off to play. Hameed looked at me and said, "I need to talk to you about something important." His face red, sweat forming on his forehead. He moved to kneel on the floor in front of me, but this was no romantic movie. He was fidgeting. He reached to hold my hands; he was shaking. He looked into my eyes and continued...

"I'm in great danger. The government is looking for me. They have arrested some of our people, and one of them betrayed the whole group."

As he explained the situation, I felt sick to my stomach. I had been afraid of this moment for so long. We were both activists fighting for our country's freedom since the new government took over in 1978. We knew the danger was imminent. We had talked about what to do in case one of us got captured.

Now, listening to this possibility becoming a probability for Hameed, I chilled. I experienced capture twelve years before when I was nineteen years old. I survived the terror of being tortured even though I was beaten so badly that I went into a coma.

So, the thought of losing the love of my life was unbearable. Our son was four years old, and I was seven months pregnant with our second child. I wanted to live with my husband, the only man I had ever loved, and the father of my children, but I knew that because of the children, I could not flee Iran. And because of the fascist regime, Hameed could not stay. I knew I had to be strong for my family. I believed I had to sacrifice my safety and happiness to save my husband's.

Hameed's brother, Reza, and his sister, Maryam, were already living in the United States. Hameed and I discussed that evening that the best way to help him was to allow him escape to America. Later I would learn that he had already discussed this with his family without my knowledge. My husband's betrayal of me began long before I joined him in Oregon.

That night, I thought I was begging him to make the difficult, but correct, decision. "You must go, Hameed. We have no other options," I demanded with tears in my eyes. "I would rather have you alive and safe but far away than dead here."

"But I don't know how long it may take before you and the kids could join me. I am not even sure I can get to America safely. What if after everything we do and plan, I still get captured? Are you sure you are up to this, Soodabeh?" Hameed seemed worried to leave me behind even though he knew we had no other choice.

I knew I had to be strong and support him, or I would lose my husband forever. So, I decided to stay behind and let Hameed escape. I was hopeful to be able to reunite with him in America soon.

No Longer Asleep but Still Imprisoned

The sound of the bathroom door closing brought me to reality. Every day, when I heard Hameed begin to move about, I started breakfast. It would be on the table, and I would be back in my chair, by the time he came into the kitchen. Without speaking, he would eat, finish, and leave the room as if I had not been sitting across from him that whole time. This day, as he finished, I spoke.

"Hameed, I don't know what is wrong with you, but I can't stand it anymore. You need to tell me what is happening, please. After everything I did for our family and saving your life by letting you escape Iran, you owe me that much."

I had never been good at confronting others, especially when I was sure the response would be bad news. My body reacted in that old way, shaking, my heart thudding. But I felt strong and rooted in those words. I had the truth on my side. He would have been killed in Iran, had I not made his leaving possible by staying behind to work and raise our children, all within the toxic space of my family home.

Hameed looked at me, finally. I could see his eyes were red, and his face had become pale, as if the blood had left his veins. He was surprised that I had demanded an answer. I took strength from that too.

"I didn't want to tell you this, but you keep pushing me. I love and care for you, but I am not in love with you anymore. I have been thinking about this for a long time. I am not crazy; I don't want to give you a false hope, thinking we are together. I hope you understand." He spoke firmly, but gently.

I knew he was talking, but I couldn't hear anything. I felt frozen, yet dizzy, and unable to feel my body from head to toe. Shortly after, I realized I could move. I got up, walked into the living room, and lay down on the cold floor. I felt my heart stop beating, yet I could still see Hameed, sitting there - so was I dead or alive?

Hameed stood up, sighed in my direction and put his dishes in the sink before leaving the apartment.

I pressed my palms against the floor. I hadn't had high expectations, just to have a roof over my head, a small room I could call my own, and to live happily with the man I had loved for many years - my husband - and the father of my children. But I realized, suddenly, sharply, that it had been a luxury to wish for that alone. Because without Hameed, this place was yet another prison. I had no other family or friends here. I did not have money or a way of earning it. I could not speak the language. I thought the deaths of my father a few years ago and then my brother only two months before I left Iran were the worst heartaches I would experience, but I was wrong.

I knew going back to Iran was completely out of the question. I had severed those ties. Besides, I couldn't bear to hurt my children. They deserved to be with their father.

I felt hopeless. The thought of living with Hameed knowing he didn't love me was unbearable. The thought of living without him, seemed impossible. *Oh, dear God, who is going to take care of me now?*

After crying for hours, I called Hameed's sister, Maryam, and told her the story. She was the only other person I knew here. I had to reach out for some help. I felt so lost that any guidance was better than none at all.

"Please, tell me what to do!" I begged my husband's sister to clue me in to his thinking. "Why did he bring me here if he didn't love me? Why did no one bother to tell me?"

"I am sorry, Soodabeh; I had no idea, I swear. He never mentioned anything. He wanted to leave my house to have a place of his own by the time you got here. He seemed very excited and happy," Maryam explained over the phone. "My house is always open to you and the kids. You have nothing to worry about. Why don't you come to stay with us for a while until we figure things out?"

I swallowed hard and scrubbed at my tear-stained face with the heels of my hands. Her offer was generous yet also led me to burst into tears again. The last time I lived with family it had been difficult, to say the least.

Shelter, Not a Home

When Hameed left Iran, the children and I moved into a small, two-bedroom apartment with my mom, and two brothers. There was no privacy or peaceful moment – for any of us. Everyone was upset all the time because of the noise of the kids fighting and crying. There was a dark cloud of desperation over all of us.

My mother and brothers hadn't signed up for this life. It was supposed to be mine, but they were forced to live the nightmare with me. I didn't want to be there either. I was working fifteen days in a row with one day off every month. With Hameed away, I needed to make money for us and for our eventual move. Plus, I thought working so much was the best way to allow my family to have some peace and quiet. The kids were in day care till I picked them up every night. I cried myself to sleep every night wishing I were with my husband.

My mother's house was our primary residence, but my toddler, newborn, and I sometimes changed residence too.

We feared being captured if we stayed in one place the whole time. Sometimes, we lived with my mother- in-law, sometimes with my sister-in-law, then back at my mother's house again.

Now, in the States, I was both tired of living with others to be safe and missing the love and support of my father and brother. I had lost my brother, Soson, to a car accident two months before I left Iran. He was a year and a half younger than me; twenty-eight at the time I was trying to leave Iran. He was a wonderful husband, son, brother, and an amazing father to his four-year-old son. At the time of his death, his wife was seven months pregnant. It was exactly the same situation as when Hameed left for America three years before; Hameed and I also had one son and I was pregnant with our second child.

"Once you settle down there, I will come to join you. I want to provide a better life for my family in freedom too," Soson had told me many times. He was there for me and my family when Hameed wasn't. He always made sure I had everything I needed and bought lots of toys for Cyrus, my son, and spent time playing with him so that he wouldn't miss his father.

Soson was my protector, my supporter, and the best brother any woman could have wished to have. He was going to help me go to the American embassy in Turkey to get the visa required to migrate to America.

I saw Soson the night before he passed away. I asked him if he was ready to accompany us to Turkey. I needed a man to go with me, but it was nerve-wracking waiting for him to get his passport in order.

"The next time you see me, I'll have my passport, and we'll go!" he said then he closed the door behind him. That was the last time I saw my sweet brother. He died the next day.

I ached for myself, losing my brother, and for my mother, losing such an incredible son. He used to call our mom several times a day, to make sure she didn't need anything.

How can I leave now? Mom just lost a son. How could she tolerate losing me too? I was angry at God for taking Soson instead of me. I had no reason to live with all this pain and agony. *Why Soson and not me, God?* I had no answers. I also knew I had to move through my grief quickly. It wasn't about me any longer; I was concerned about the rest of our family.

Mom had lost her husband, my father, to a sudden heart attack when he was forty-seven. I was the oldest of five. At that time, I was thirteen with three brothers. Soson, eleven; Soheil, six; and Seamak, only two years old. My parents had adopted a girl, my age, named Maggy, when her parents died in an earthquake.

My father was a wonderful, kind, and loving man. He always tried to talk gently to us kids. Although he hadn't graduated from high school, he was very intelligent, and loved reading books about everything and anything: history, geography, psychology, philosophy, and even religion. In the local café, he and many college students used to gather to discuss what he had read. At times, my father would even help the students with their assignments.

At home, I remember he would join us children on the floor with a small table full of books in front of him and many more volumes all around him on the carpet. If the book he was reading referenced a second book, Dad would buy the other book to read it too. My father was easily able to quote from every book he had read.

"What are you doing, Dad?" I would ask.

"Oh, hey, honey, come sit by me, and I will show you. Try to see if you can read this sentence for me, baby."

His eyes shone with joy and excitement, watching me read. Do you understand what they are talking about?" he would ask.

"Not really, Dad," I would respond, laughing.

"Well, it means…" And he would explain in detail.

My father didn't complete high school because he too lost his father at a young age. My grandfather died when my dad was only sixteen years old, leaving my grandmother with two young children. My grandparents had many children, but they all died, except two; my dad and his younger sister. My grandmother was unable to work since women didn't work outside of the home in those days. Consequently, my father had to quit school and go to work to support his family. He loved and adored his mother and sister. He would do anything they wanted without complaint; It was in his nature to help and please others.

Hopeless

Oh, how much I miss you Dad. I thought now. *I wish I had you and Soson with me now. Oh, God, I can't live like this.*

Looking back at my life in Iran for the past three years, I realized that, although it was extremely challenging, at least I was able to speak the language. I had a job, and the support of my family and friends. The thought of living alone and trying to take care of my family in America was horrifying. I had never lived alone. And I had never been able to make decisions alone, even when I was in Iran. Furthermore, I was unable to return to Iran – I'd be in danger there, and my children would be without their father.

I also still loved Hameed, in spite of everything he had said and done. I wanted him so desperately; I needed him. I began hoping Hameed would come to his senses. I would have to wait until Shahab, Maryam's husband, picked me and the children up after his work day ended.

It was late in the evening when Shahab came knocking on the door. Hameed was in the bedroom sleeping. Cyrus and Azeeta, my daughter, were barely awake, lying on the sofa watching TV quietly. I had already packed our suitcases. With a heavy heart, I stood up to open the door and welcomed Shahab to come in.

"Are you guys ready?" he asked, reaching out to hold Azeeta in his arms, then he kissed her forehead. "Come on. Let's go sweetheart."

Shahab lit a cigarette at the bottom of the porch stairs after dragging our two heavy suitcases down there. Adjusting his glasses, he exhaled, smoke coming out of his mouth and nostrils. He put the cigarette between his lips, bent his six-foot frame at the waist, and picked up the suitcases, again resuming the walk toward his car. After putting them inside the trunk, he continued to smoke, leaning backward against the car, and waiting for me to get the kids settled in the car. He dropped the cigarette on the ground, stepped on it, got inside the car, and started driving toward his house.

Cyrus and Azeeta were quiet, their faces pale with the anguish over what they had witnessed and leaving their father. Every time I felt the tears well up, I wiped at my eyes, trying to hide them from the kids. I wasn't sure why –I'd been crying a lot in front of them recently, but to keep my sadness private was still in my nature.

I had known Maryam for over thirteen years. She was my best friend and supporter. Although I knew I could trust her, Hameed was her brother. Hameed was the youngest of seven, and Maryam was two years older than him. They had been very close since childhood, and I knew she would do anything for him. I had a feeling it would be difficult and challenging to live there. I didn't expect her to take our side and stay away from Hameed. I knew that would be impossible.

When we finally arrived after twenty silent minutes, Maryam invited us in, but her smile looked cold and fake. She didn't reach out to hug any of us and never looked me in the eyes.

"Please be quiet," she whispered. "The kids are sleeping. They have to wake up early to go to school tomorrow."

On her tiptoes, she guided us to the kids' bedroom where a queen-size mattress had been added on the floor. It was covered with white sheets, three white pillows, and a few beige woolen blankets. Her kids, Jake, and Sam continued sleeping in their beds.

Maryam left, closing the door behind her, but I could hear her and Shahab whispering. I had a gut feeling Hameed might have called her before we got there.

I tried to quiet my mind and go to sleep, but I couldn't. I felt my life was over. I had no one to go to. I had no one to talk with. I didn't have the heart to call my mother and tell her what Hameed had done. I was ashamed of my situation even though I knew it wasn't my fault. I had endured so much already, from being tortured into a coma to losing my father and my brother, to now losing my husband. I felt I was doomed for life; I felt stuck with no way out.

There is no hope. No one can help me. I can't go on without Hameed. I just can't. I don't want to live anymore. This is the end for me.

Reader, my friend, what I'm about to tell you next may seem so irrational that it couldn't have happened. At that moment, while lying on the floor, listening to that relentless rain pound against the windows, I made a plan to end my life that night.

I don't see any reason to live. I don't know why God didn't take me instead of Soson. No one can help me. There is no hope. I am done.

You are right that this thinking makes no sense. There were so many paths for me, even in that terrible moment. At the least, you may think, I should have been thinking of my children and figured something out, for their sake! But if you are reading this book, I also know that you understand irrational thinking. Many of us will reach a point in life when we find ourselves within a tunnel and cannot see the light at the end of it. The tunnel becomes a cave, with a rock rolling to cover its exit.

That night, feeling ashamed, guilty, and with a heavy heart, the children sleeping beside me, I got out of bed. The house was noticeably quiet. Even the rain had ceased, as though the sky were holding its breath. I could hear my heart beating in my chest. I closed the bedroom door behind me and walked down the narrow, dark hallway into the dining room. I slowly picked up a chair and tiptoed into the kitchen. I stepped onto the dark brown chair, and tried to keep my balance as I reached to open the cupboard over my head.

I am sure Hameed will take care of the kids. He has a brother and a sister here. I know they will help him to raise the kids. It's better if I don't exist.

I found a couple of over-the-counter pain relievers. I pried open the lids and was disappointed to discover that there were only a few pills in each.

This must be my luck, fewer than ten pills. I am sure it's not even enough to knock me out, but maybe it will work. I picked up a glass, filled it with tap water, and swallowed all the pills at once.

I walked back into the bedroom and lay down between Cyrus and Azeeta.

I love you. I hope you forgive me someday. I know I am not being a good mother by going out this way. I am sorry, sweethearts.

I kissed both their faces and tried to sleep, praying to never wake up. I felt guilty leaving them behind, but I still believed their lives would be less of a mess without me.

"Mom, Mom, wake up"

I felt my son Cyrus shaking my arms.

I am alive? I can't believe this. Why can't I open my eyes, then?

"Wait, honey," I told Cyrus with slurred speech. "Please... I am tryyying to ... – get up. Pleasssse, stop - shaking meee. I have a — headache." It was as though I were cast in stone. I tried to cover my face with the blanket, hoping Cyrus would leave me alone.

Cyrus and Azeeta scampered away and a minute later, I heard my sister-in-law say, her voice rising, so I would hear her. "Go wake up your mother. This is not a hotel. We don't have room service here."

Suddenly, I was flesh and blood and bone again. I almost threw up as I stood – the room was spinning faster than I could breathe. I hoped to faint and hit my head, but I stayed alert.

I had tried to end my life but failed miserably. I was angry at God for taking so many people I loved. I was angry at myself for being saved so many times.

Hope

Reader, I suspect you have been in a situation similar to mine. Trying to get back up after losing a loved one, a relationship, or a job. Maybe life just feels really difficult and you've come to the end of your wits and patience with it all.

But I'm saying to you, from twenty-nine years after my lowest moment, that no matter where you are in life, you need to know you have the power to change the outcome. You have the power to choose which direction to go. You are never hopeless or helpless.

Sharing my story, I want to inspire you to believe in miracles – miracles created by you when you set boundaries, quit with the excuses, shame, guilt, and blame, and use the power you already have to be better, do better, and find peace within.

Believe me when I say that you have more than what I had twenty-nine years ago. You can speak the language. You know where to go, who to talk to for help. We live in the internet age. You can search for and find every answer; you can even ask your mom, best friend or your old teacher, because they are just an email or a video call away even if they live far away.

But ultimately, while you should seek help, the answer is not outside you. Just as you are the only one who can *break* you, you are the only one who can *help* you. You are the only one who can rescue you and love you unconditionally.

No one will care for you if you don't care for yourself first. No one will support you if you don't first support yourself. You are the master and creator of your life. You have the power to create your destiny. Stop believing the lies you were told while growing up. Stop believing that you are not good enough, young enough, tall enough, or smart enough.

I grew up feeling that I never belonged. I was different from all my family. I was told by many family members, friends, and even co-workers that I wasn't enough because I was short. I was told I wasn't allowed to decide, so I was unable to make decisions for myself. I was weak in the face of my family's high expectations, so I had no self-esteem or confidence of any sort. I was no one without my family, and I was no one without my husband.

I grew up with my mother doing everything for me and having my husband take over that role after I got married. I lived dependent on others until life put me in a situation where I was forced to live alone, to make decisions for my family, and to be the only one who could love and care for me.

And then this really exciting thing happened: once I realized I could do that, and once I did do that, suddenly, I had many strangers in this foreign land come to my aid. I learned to help myself, but I did not stand alone.

My neighbors (once I started smiling as I passed them), my classmates and teachers (once I enrolled in school to prepare to make a living), and strangers (once I shared my story with authenticity so that they could see themselves in there too) all offered helping hands, food and clothes for my family.

I woke up every day reminding myself to breathe, to take a shower, to walk a few more steps, to go outside, to talk to people even though I didn't know the language.

And to my surprise, people opened their arms and their big hearts, and they tried to understand me patiently. They listened; they paid attention to me. They offered help and assistance I never thought was possible. Ask and you shall receive. I prayed day and night. And I was grateful for every living, breathing person who came into my life.

So, if you are feeling hopeless, if you feel you have no choice, think again. The possibilities are endless when you decide to live, to love, to forgive, to take responsibility, and to be accountable for creating the life you want and deserve. We all are gifted individuals. We are different, but the Creator has blessed us with certain gifts, talents, dreams.

I realized long after my low point, almost thirty years ago, that more than a husband, a home and the love of others, what I was desperately seeking at that time was answers. And all the answers were inside me, found by me, with the support of others. I hope this book is one of your guides.

Food for Thought

What crossroads are you standing at?

What's a truly terrifying situation you experienced? Did you survive?

Have you experienced a challenge you didn't expect? Did you discover you had prepared for it without realizing it, or what did you do to rise to meet that challenge?

Have you let yourself grieve?

Have you blamed God for something? Have you found the true source of your anguish, and how did you do that?

What's a blessing in your life? Think of one, even if everything feels dark, and it has to be the tiniest of good things.

I am here if you need help. All you need to do is to reach out. Email, call, or have a quick consultation with me. I will show you the way.

www.soodabehmokry.com

Chapter Two

Step One: Acknowledge and Accept Where You Are

I knew that although I hated being alive, I had to find a solution. And living with Maryam was not it. I knew Maryam didn't want me there; the feeling was mutual. I knew I couldn't ask her to be in the middle and choose me over her brother. It wasn't fair to any of us. I realized that I had no choice but to acknowledge my situation. I picked up the phone and begged Hameed to come and take me home. I didn't care about anything else, but grieving in my own space.

"Please come take us home. I don't want to live like this. I am tired. I need a break," I cried over the phone.

"Are you sure you want to come back? You know nothing will change, right?"

"I don't care. Just get me out of here. I would rather be by myself now."

"Can you at least stay there until I get off work?" Hameed said before hanging up the phone.

I tried to keep Cyrus and Azeeta busy even though I felt dizzy, sick, and tired. I sat them on the couch to watch TV until Hameed came to pick us up. He dragged our big suitcases, lifting them up and put them in the trunk of his car before driving us back to the apartment. It was late in the evening, a dark and wet night from raining all day.

We had already eaten dinner at Maryam's and the kids were tired. I helped them change into their pajamas and tucked them in bed. I lay down on the bed next to Azeeta, wishing Hameed would get up from where he was sitting in the living room watching TV and come and hold me in his arms.

I woke up the next morning to the sound of the front door closing; Hameed had left for work. I wished I had a friend to talk with. I wished I could call my family and ask for advice. But I couldn't because I was ashamed.

As though my anxious thoughts had become a prayer, I suddenly thought of someone I could call: Shahab, Maryam's husband who had defended me. Shahab loved my children as his own. Shahab was like a brother to me. He knew I was grieving the loss of my brother. He knew I was alone and suffering. I thought maybe he would have an answer.

I picked up the phone, "I am sorry to bother you," I said when I heard my brother-in-law's voice, "but I can't live like this anymore. I am miserable, and so are my children. What do you think is going to happen to us now?"

Shahab's voice was gentle. "I can't believe Hameed is doing this. I don't know what is wrong with that man. He has gone crazy, I swear. Please don't worry. I will come to visit after work this evening."

As I hung up, I noticed Cyrus by my side. He was angry. "It's all your fault, Mom," he said. His tiny voice cut me like the sharpest blade. "Why can't you stop fighting with my dad?"

I had heard the desperation in his voice many times before. Cyrus loved his father. He had tolerated a lot of anguish over three years in the hope of one day living again with his father. He had no idea what I was going through. He was too young to understand. And I had no idea how to fix it.

"Cyrus, believe me, I am fighting to keep your dad from leaving."

"Then stop fighting *with* him. Stop making him leave every time he comes home."

Our job as parents is to protect our children from harm. We try to do the best we can to keep them safe, so they don't get hurt. We try to create a safe place for them, so they will be happy and joyful while growing up. I had the same intention in every step I took; every effort was to protect them from knowing the truth about their father not wanting to be around, but I had failed miserably.

I felt like the worst mother, and I wished Cyrus would comprehend what I had done for them.

Later that evening, Shahab knocked on the door. Azeeta ran to the door upon hearing his voice. "Open the door!" she cried, too little to turn the knob herself. "It's Uncle Shahab."

Relieved as I saw that Shahab was there, this moment reminded me that, at a very early age, Azeeta didn't know who her father was. Although Hameed loved her, the turmoil of our living situation for the past few weeks had prevented them from bonding as they should have. Remember, my friend, Hameed left Iran before Azeeta was born.

Shahab sat on the couch across from me. It had been a long day for him working for ten hours, and he hadn't even gone home yet. He cared about our situation and was trying to help.

"Listen to me," he said. "You don't deserve to live like this. No one does. It's up to you to decide about your future. Hameed has not done anything for you or the kids. Is this how you want to live; depending on him forever?"

"But I don't have money, I can't speak English, and I don't know how to get anywhere. How am I going to survive without Hameed?"

"What has he done for you so far? Has he taken you anywhere? Has he tried to show you the city? Has he taught you English? Has he found a job for you? Tell me, please, I am listening. Why can't you live without him?" he was speaking firmly, but gently, so the kids didn't hear him.

My heart was aching with the worst pain I had ever experienced knowing Shahab was right. I had allowed fear to prevent me from seeing the truth. Yet, still I fought against myself. I wanted to believe in the impossible rather than trying to accept the truth.

"Hameed said he would help me to go to school and find a job."

"When? He hasn't done anything but fight with you for the past month since you arrived. You are an intelligent, hardworking woman. You have worked and raised your kids without him so far, haven't you? If you don't want to think about yourself, at least consider your children. This is not right or fair for them to suffer. You need to wake up, Soodabeh!"

"Yes, you are right, but I am scared. I have never lived alone, even when I was in Iran. I lived with my family. I don't know what to do, how to make decisions alone without anyone's help. I am really scared, Shahab." My body shook uncontrollably, and I burst into tears.

"You are in America, the land of opportunities. You will have help and assistance, I promise you. I will be there for you. I will never leave you and the kids alone," he continued. "But you must decide and start now. You will wake up and regret your decision if you stay with him. Believe me, every day counts. If you wait a day, you may fall behind a year. You can get loans, financial aid, and go to school. You were a nurse in Iran, and I am sure you can do the same here. But it is your call."

"Maryam told me it's difficult to go to school here. I don't know the language. Hameed said the nursing school is very challenging too."

I kept throwing up roadblocks, but deep down I knew Shahab was right. I had to accept my situation. Hameed was not coming back, and I knew it would be a waste of time waiting for him. I had wasted three years waiting for him already. I had endured the most challenging living situation possible in Iran. The more I listened to Shahab, who so patiently kept knocking down every complaint and fear as soon as I had erected it, the more convinced I felt, believing I was strong and capable of doing anything.

Hameed arrived as Shahab was getting ready to leave. "What are you doing here?" Hameed asked, not angry but surprised.

"I am sorry. I don't want to come between you two, but I think it's better if you guys separate from each other and move on with your lives," Shahab said, standing up tall. "Hameed, you need to let her go, let her move on if you really don't want her."

Shahab looked at me, his hand on the doorknob, and said one more time in front of Hameed. "What do you want to do, Soodabeh? It's your decision." And then Shahab left.

I collapsed on the sofa after putting the kids to bed. Hameed sat on the coffee table, leaning toward me, and after he adjusted his glasses, he looked in my eyes and said, gently, "I have decided to go live with a friend. That way, you can have the apartment. I have already paid the rent for December and will pay for next month, too. I don't need anything except my clothes. You can keep the apartment as long as you pay the rent. You can get public assistance- the money won't be much, but it will be enough for the rent on this small apartment. You don't have a car, and you cook at home, so your expenses are small."

I was on my knees. My blubbering frustrated him. Hameed interjected, "I can't live with you anymore. I promise to help you to get a job and get your life together, but I can't live with you. Stop begging, please... Just stop!"

My intuition had warned me about this, but I had refused to believe Hameed would ever leave me. When I was still in Iran, I had a dream he was with another woman. Everything was making sense now. My nightmare had come true. No matter what I said and did, nothing would fix our broken relationship. I had to decide. I had to choose.

With tears in my eyes and a heavy heart, I began packing Hameed's clothes in one of my suitcases and finally said goodbye to the man I had loved for years. I knew the dream of living with him as my husband and the father of my children was just a fantasy.

Hameed left without saying goodbye this time. It was different. It was real. My marriage was over this time. No more hugs, no more kisses like he did three years ago when leaving Iran. This time he was not coming back.

Cyrus and Azeeta were sleeping in bed. I sat on the couch and sobbed uncontrollably. Life had forced me to finally grow up. I had to acknowledge my situation and accept that I had choices, but in that, I also could believe I had the power of choice. I got to decide. I could choose to either be miserable and wait for Hameed to come back someday, when I knew he wouldn't, or I could choose to move on without him. I had the power to make the best decision for our family. I was being given the ultimate choice: to do or die. I had tried to die but failed. Now, I had to choose another way. I had to choose to live.

I had to accept my situation. I had to decide to try to find other solutions. If Shahab was right, then I had a better life waiting for me. I had to have faith in my ability to make the right decision. What was I going to lose?

I needed to begin thinking differently. It wasn't just about me and my life. It was about my children. I had promised them a better life. I was obligated to do what I had promised to do. I had to make the first and most crucial decision of my lifetime, alone. That night, I decided to choose my happiness for once.

I was frightened not knowing what my life would be like, but I knew the first step to creating a better life was to simply let Hameed go!

If You Wait a Day, You May Fall Behind a Year

Acknowledging where you are is the most important step to finding a solution. You can't deny the situation and hope to have a better outcome. You can't repeat the same thing every day and expect a different result.

We all have choices – that's what this book is about. It's our mindset that keeps us stuck. Our limited thoughts and beliefs about our ability to be and do more prevent us from taking actions. (I will discuss mindset in detail in chapter four). Something deep within me changed the minute I decided to acknowledge and accept that Hameed wasn't coming back. Acceptance of my situation made me look for solutions- the next step- with a new mindset. It helped me to keep moving forward in hope of creating a better life for my family.

We are always in control of our feelings and emotions. What we do with our challenging situation is the key to success. I had the choice of not accepting my situation and staying in that miserable frame of mind- thinking and hoping Hameed would come back one day. Trust me, I have met people over the years who feel stuck and resentful, expecting more from life.

They say, "I have no choice." I believed this at first too, but that's just an illusion that the mind is trying to convince us is real. The truth is that we do have many choices and are capable of choosing if we want to.

Believe me, I am not going to lie and tell you that having the power of choice will feel like a blessing at first. It does not. It's hard, and it's challenging. It's scary not being able to see the end result. Happiness didn't happen overnight for me, and it won't happen quickly for you either. That's why they call it *faith*; because you move forward trusting you are on the right path even when you cannot see or even comprehend what will happen next.

Being stuck with the feelings of shame, guilt, and blame only stops you from creating the most magnificent life, family, relationship, finances, and business. It will take you away from the truth of being the powerful and creative spirit you were born to be. The everyday negative thoughts and beliefs you are dealing with, often marked by questions such as "why?" and 'what if', will prevent you from bringing the magic and synchronicity into your daily experiences.

I remember many years ago I met a beautiful woman... let's call her Judy. She was tall and gorgeous. She had long blond hair and beautiful blue eyes. To me, she was one of the most beautiful women I had ever met. She had a great life ahead of her, but she was sad and filled with anger. Her husband had left her many years before and had chosen a different life. Judy had custody of their children, but her husband was taking care of her financially and supporting the children.

In my mind, she should have been happy and able to create a life of her own. She had every opportunity in life to do something that would make her happy. But for many years, almost a decade in fact, she chose to be angry, resentful, and stuck. "I don't feel any desire to go out or try to date. I like being home alone and staying in my world," she explained.

There are many people who are happy and content living alone. I was well aware of this fact. As an introvert, I have always loved my quiet time at home. Being happy doesn't necessarily mean being in a relationship. I have chosen not to date and am happy and content with the life I have created. But that was my choice based on self-love, not on anger or low self-esteem.

Judy was angry and resentful regarding her past relationship. She was unhappy not being in a meaningful relationship. Judy was unable to move forward and enjoy life. She had chosen fear and anger instead of joy and peace. I felt sad for her and the way she chose to live. She kept blaming her ex-husband for what he did over ten years earlier and refused to do anything to feel fulfilled in her own life. Judy was unable to acknowledge and accept her situation. She was lost in the negative memories of her past. I knew Judy had the power to choose to feel better, be successful, and enjoy her life if she wanted to, but she chose differently. I wished she would find her way out of the darkness soon.

In another story, I remember caring for one of my patients who was a medical professional. He was having a difficult time accepting the outcome of his illness. Let's call him John for the sake of revealing this story.

John was a prominent professional in his field and had a highly successful life before he became ill. John survived the exceedingly difficult journey of cancer and was in the recovery process. However, in order to save John's life, the doctor removed a part of his intestine causing him to have a colostomy bag and a large open wound in his stomach. My job as a nurse was to go to his home and teach him and his wife how to care for the colostomy and to do wound care. John's abdominal wound was not healing in spite of everything we tried. John was soft spoken and a gentle soul, but he was upset dealing with the loss of his independence and facing a situation he had no control over.

It is normal to feel angry when experiencing any loss. It's a part of the journey to go through different stages of grief. Sometimes we are able to move through each stage easily, and sometimes we get stuck in a stage. I knew his healing process wouldn't progress because John wasn't willing to accept his situation.

I knew I had to be honest with John in the most compassionate and loving way possible to help him to move forward. One day as I was visiting him, I saw him very frustrated at the fact that his wound wasn't healing.

"What am I doing wrong? Why does it have to be this way?" John expressed, raising his voice at the situation.

"John, with all due respect, as long as you feel angry and resentful for having a colostomy, and refuse to make peace with it, your wound will not heal."

I wasn't sure how he would react to what I had said, but I saw his expression soften up as he looked at me.

"What did you just say?" he said gently, but he didn't need me to repeat myself. "I think you are right, Soodabeh. How can I do that? How can I accept this bag that smells all the time? No matter how many times I take a shower, I can still smell it. I am afraid to go back to work. I am ashamed when people come close to me. I can't stop feeling this way."

I knew what I said allowed him to express what he had felt for months. We live in a society that prevents men from expressing their emotions. He was raised to be strong and independent. He was a key person in his family and career, always helping and taking care of others. He didn't know how to care about himself.

"John, no one smells this but you. The issue is that your mind is making you believe that something is wrong with your situation. Trust me, as long as you fight with this and dwell on what is rather than accepting it, your wound will not heal. Healing your body can't happen if your mind negates and believes something is wrong. You need to make peace with your situation. Your wife and your family love you the same if not more now. Are you ready to be willing today to try to accept your situation? You just have to accept it one day at a time."

He listened. Then he accepted his healing one step at a time. It was amazing the way his wound became smaller and smaller every day; he healed faster than anyone thought was possible. Every time I would visit, he would look at me with pride knowing that he was contributing to his well-being and healing. He was discharged shortly after he decided to accept his situation.

Accepting the situation prevents you from feeling stuck, or looking backward and trying to figure out why or what went wrong. You need to accept what has been done and focus on your next step of creating the best life possible. Learn the lesson and move forward. I know, it's not easy at times.

When the emotions arise to surface, acknowledge them, and let them go. You need to be able to redirect your mind to accepting what is. Some days are easier than others, but you must be consistent. You must be focused on what you want to create in your journey. You can still grieve for what you had, but accepting what is, opens the doors of creativity and aspirations awaiting to come into your everyday reality. (You will learn more about the tools and how to redirect your mind in detail in chapter five.)

Growing up in a culture where women had to be submissive and always ready to serve their husband and family, I learned to discount my feelings and emotions. If I had a hard day and felt upset about something, I would immediately start beating myself up for getting upset. I was taught to always be happy and cheerful to accommodate others. Self-care didn't have any room in my upbringing at all.

I learned this the hard way. After many years of feeling ashamed, guilty, and trying to resist my own feelings, I realized one day that the best thing I could do was to accept how I felt. On one particularly tough day, whatever had happened earlier brought the negative emotions of my past experiences. I realized something within me became activated in a different way. Instead of being upset about my own feelings, I began giving myself permission to feel whatever was bothering me.

I knew I had experienced a lot, and my mind and body were exhausted, asking me to have compassion, love, and understanding for myself. These were strange words in my vocabulary. I would get upset with myself because I was feeling sad remembering the past. I was trying to resist the feeling because it was painful to experience the emotions over and over again. I had no idea these feelings and emotions had come to surface because they needed to be acknowledged and healed in order for me to truly move forward in life.

I remember what I said. Like a lion roaring in the wild, I felt the words blurt out of my mouth without my control. "I have been through a lot in my life. So if today, and for whatever reason, I am upset, I have the right to feel that way. I have the right to be upset and angry. I have the right to be me, with my feelings, in the privacy of my home."

I had no idea where that thought and the words were coming from, but I could hear them loud and clear from within me. I went about my day, and after about an hour, I didn't feel upset anymore. Normally when I would get upset, it would linger for a day or two. But this time was different. I suddenly realized from this experience that, when we accept and embrace our emotions rather than resisting or dwelling over them, the feelings will pass quickly.

I was amazed how it worked like magic. I had no idea about this process, no one had taught me, I just followed the thought, or I should say the intuitive guidance to embrace the situation. (I will discuss the concept of intuition in chapter six). I had allowed myself to sit in the pain. I had allowed myself to grieve. And then I had allowed myself to let go. I learned I was human and can't always be cheerful and happy. I learned that accepting the difficult and unpleasant emotions as a human being is normal and natural. I realized I needed to stop beating myself up for feeling sad, lonely, or upset about something.

I have used this easy technique of *embracing your emotions* with my clients for many years now. I have seen improvement in their journey of overcoming life challenges when dealing with their emotions. Honor your emotions and express your feelings rather than feeling consumed by shame and guilt about why you feel a certain way. It takes time to overcome feelings of loss. However, acknowledging and accepting your situation allows you to get to the next stage of your journey more quickly. You may go back and forth through the stages of grief, trying to figure out what happened at times. You may feel shocked, experience blame or denial at some points; these feelings are a normal part of the grief process.

Remember to just be gentle with yourself. Acknowledge the feelings, sit with them without judging why you feel the way you do. Treat and comfort yourself the way you would a sorrowful friend. We don't judge others when they are experiencing life challenges, right? Have the same love and compassion for yourself to get through your day.

Do One Thing

Here are things I used to do:

- I stayed in unhealthy relationships due to the fear of being alone for the rest of my life.

- I worked in unethical companies because I was afraid I would never find a better job.

- I didn't want to acknowledge there was an issue because admitting to myself there was something wrong meant that I had to make a decision to fix the situation.

- I spent money because the act of shopping made me feel like I had purpose.

- I chose to eat excessively as a way to feel better about my situation.

- I ate and watched TV mindlessly, trying to get lost in that story, so I didn't feel so lost in my own.

Are these examples making sense to you? I hope it's helping to know that you are not alone. Accept your situation and do your best to go forward through life. No more blaming, no more victimhood, no more delving deep into addictions, and no more excuses. Addictions could be about food, alcohol, shopping, drugs, sex, gambling, or even TV. You are a good person trying to feel comfort in the wrong way, dear one. There is a better life waiting for you. And you are the one who has to choose.

When feelings come to surface, acknowledge, accept, and move forward. I have noticed that reading uplifting books and watching or listening to inspiring stories has always helped to take me to a higher level mentally and emotionally. Doing these things makes me feel more positive and optimistic. Or try joining a support group, hiring a coach, or attending counseling. Sometimes being with a group of people who share similar experiences allows you to not feel alone in your journey and helps you to move up from where you are.

Need more information?

Visit my website at: http://www.soodabehmokry.com/

Email me: info@soodabehmokry.com

Or

Join my FB group:
https://www.facebook.com/groups/globalholistichealing/

Chapter Three

Step two: Decide What You Want

In order to move forward in life, I had to make sure my decisions were positive and rewarding. I was the only one in charge of me. Going to school to learn English as a second language while Cyrus was at school and Azeeta was at the babysitter was the next step for me. I was excited to take steps toward creating my new life. I felt elated to wake up every day knowing I would be taking care of myself.

At times, my heart was filled with grief, trying to figure out where Hameed was and what he was doing. Was he thinking about me? But I learned there was a better way and that was to focus on what I had in front of me rather than focusing on the past.

I had survived life so far. I knew there would be something better waiting for me. My faith in God and the love I had for my children encouraged me to wake up every morning with hope and the desire to do something different.

Guides Among Us

My first day of school was nerve-wracking because I didn't know the language. However, getting to know many people from all over the world who also didn't know the language was comforting. It's amazing that kindness and unconditional love shine through even when we aren't able to otherwise understand one another. Smiles and the attempts to start a conversation were pure and joyful.

Gradually, I noticed people had been chosen to be my guides to help me to go to the next stage of my life. In Iran, when someone decided to move and do something about their life, we would tell them that God would intervene and help them by opening the right doors. I had hopes and dreams and was about to witness God's help and guidance every step.

I had classmates who became my friends. They helped me and my family by taking us grocery shopping, and providing clothes for my children who were quickly growing. I talk more in-depth about these amazing people in my first book, *Angel Nightingale*. They were my angels in physical form on earth to help me survive.

I remember, my mother used to talk about my father and how he helped many people physically, emotionally, and financially. According to my mother, my father used to say that nothing he was doing would be lost in God's eyes. He was serving God's children and knew his children would never go without. I didn't understand it growing up but, being in a different country and without the support of family, I began to understand what my father had said and done.

I also knew the spirits of my father and brother were always with me. I had learned about this from childhood. We believe the spirit of our loved ones are always with us as our guardian angels. I was able to witness that every day in the way my neighbors, my children's babysitter, and my classmates showed me love and compassion. I felt God had chosen a new family for me in America; the most precious and loving family I could ever imagine having.

I had one of the most amazing English teachers as well. Melinda was kind, loving, and generous. She was always trying to find solutions outside of class to help us succeed in life. It was not a coincidence that everything in heaven and earth was lining up to help and guide me everyday. I couldn't discount this truth. That was the reason I kept going with a smile on my face. I wanted to work hard and achieve expedited success. I was reading English language books, watching American TV with my children, and speaking English at home with my children. When Melinda realized I was really focused on learning and growing faster than usual, she reached out to me even more. She asked questions about my life story and what had brought me to America. When she found out how I was left alone with two young children, she felt compassion toward me and began trying to help me even more outside of the class.

"Soodabeh, you know there are free tutors. Would you be interested?"

"Of course! I need to learn so I can start working and making money to support my children."

Every day I would hear some new information that gave me more hope and faith that I was on the right path. I had no idea how long I had and which way I would go, but I was determined and thirsty for knowledge.

One day when I was talking to Melinda, I told her about my life in Iran and how I worked as a nurse for ten years. She looked deep into my eyes, her big brown eyes beaming with the brightest light I had ever seen, while she held my hands and smiled.

"Soodabeh, do you know we have the best nursing program in this college? There is an advisor I can introduce you to so you can get more information. You can go take some classes since you were a nurse in Iran.

I went immediately to the school advisor. She pointed me further along my path. "Soodabeh," she said gently, "you can attend the nursing program and succeed after a few years. The Bridge to Success Program here is designed to help minorities succeed in school. You have a great chance here."

I thought this was definitely a divine intervention. Listening to her talking about the program and all the tools available to me was exciting. I had the chance to learn in a program created for students from different ethnic backgrounds. It was unbelievable to hear all the promising news in the first few weeks of me attending school to learn English. I could see there was definitely a better future waiting for me. I was slowly able to comprehend what Shahab had told me earlier. I knew then that he was right.

The truth is that when we decide to do whatever it takes to get our life together, magic and synchronistic events enter our reality. People come into our life for a purpose to help and guide us to the next step. This has been the case in my life for the past twenty-nine years. I can't make these things up. I am a firm believer that, when the student is ready, the teacher will show up. When we are ready and determined to do something, the Universe, God, the Divine Source will intervene. The doors of opportunities will open with minimal effort. Life becomes magic and full of pleasant surprises. Everything becomes easy and effortless taking you to the next step.

One day when Hameed came to pick up the kids, I told him about my experience at school.

"I am going to go to school and get my nursing degree," I said with excitement like a little, innocent girl.

He started laughing. "Are you serious? Do you know how difficult it is? You can't even speak English yet," he said amused.

"Why, do you think it's difficult? I am going to work hard and start the program when I am ready. I am going to be able to work as a nurse!" I replied firmly standing up with my hands on my hips filled with confidence. I looked directly into his eyes and continued, "I will show you, Hameed. Trust me, I will make it without you, I promise!"

"Listen, Soodabeh," Hameed responded, "The closest you can come to working in a hospital is to clean the toilets," he continued laughing, and then he left.

I had been listening to Hameed tell me for many years that I couldn't make decisions, or that I wasn't able to take care of myself without the help of others. I had lived every day believing I would literally die without him. But that was the last thing I needed to hear. I realized his statement about me being incapable of choosing and doing what I wanted was the fire I needed in my gut to keep going and prove him wrong. I had heard such comments from him and his sister before but, at that moment, I finally decided to refuse to believe them. Something within me was telling me otherwise.

I knew I needed to stop listening to what others said that prevented me from reaching my highest potential. I felt life had given me another chance. I felt I was born again. I had dreams and aspirations. I was alive. I realized that listening to others who didn't do anything to help me was just a waste of my time. I was determined to make it and create the most beautiful life possible for me in America. I wasn't afraid of working hard. I had worked fifteen days in a row over and over when I was a nurse in Iran.

I had raised my children while working and without any emotional or physical support from my family for three years. I had the luxury of living with my family in Iran, but I did everything else to make a living and provide for my family. I began thinking and believing that I was able to make decisions. I decided that day that I would succeed no matter what. I also realized that I had made the perfect decision to let Hameed leave. It was a new time, a new beginning. I was proud and ready to start making new decisions for my family- alone.

Finding an Outlet

I was working with two tutors, one who spoke my language, and the other one spoke English and was American. I had to do my best to prove to myself and others that I could succeed. Jeff, my American tutor, helped me not only learn English but develop my writing. He was the one who encouraged me to start writing about my life. This allowed me to express my most intimate and deepest thoughts and emotions without the fear of criticism. It was healing for me to get the words out of my system.

I used to write poems in my journal when I was a teenager growing up in Iran. That was the only way I could get my feelings out since I wasn't allowed to talk about them. My mother was extremely strict and didn't allow me to have friends. I was an introvert and didn't like to talk about my feelings anyway. Part of this issue was because of my low self-esteem. My mother and family never asked me about my thoughts or opinion regarding anything. My family were the ones who made decisions, and I was expected to follow them. I felt invisible at times growing up. I had accepted and believed that no one loved me. I realized many years later that this wasn't the case. Nevertheless, it had been true to me.

It was amazing that people in my new country liked me. They noticed me and paid attention to me. They were interested in me and what I had to say. People were asking questions and respected my thoughts and beliefs. I felt more at home here in America than when I was growing up in Iran with my family.

As I wrote and uncovered these truths, I began to understand why God had saved my life so many times. From somewhere deep within me, I could sense why my life wasn't over yet. I began to understand that I must have a purpose or a mission to still be alive after everything I had experienced. Life was wonderful and magical, and best of all- it was just the beginning.

Big Gains

After a few months, I was able to apply for financial aid. I had completed learning English as a second language and was ready to take credit classes at the college. This allowed me to be eligible to receive loans. It also afforded me the opportunity to work as an English tutor and teach the students coming from other countries who didn't know basic English. I was proud to be a mentor and grateful for the opportunity to help others while getting paid for my services. I was feeling true abundance in every area of my life- physical, emotional, and financial.

I began taking more prerequisite classes to start nursing school. I had grown into a different person, more powerful and determined than I had ever imagined. Life was amazing, rewarding, and peaceful. I didn't have to think or deal with others who didn't support me in my journey. I was independent and able to do whatever I loved to do. My children were happy to see me grow as well. Watching my children enjoying life was priceless. They had endured so much pain in the last few years.

We didn't have much. I didn't have a car or any other luxury that required payment except my rent, food and basic household items. I was living in a very small one-bedroom apartment in a low-income neighborhood. I used to make sandwiches and take my kids to the school playground to play while I would study. But with school loans, financial aid, and income from work study and babysitting, I was able to have a decent life.

More than all that, I finally had enough confidence to let my family in Iran know about my situation and divorce from Hameed. They were worried about me at first, but when they learned more about my being able to go to school to have a good life, they accepted it.

Food for Thought

I had made my decision to let Hameed go, which had led to doors of opportunity opening. Entering a new life with choices and possibilities beyond my wildest dreams was thrilling. Learning English and being able to keep a conversation with people was rewarding. Every little victory made me want to do more and take more steps toward creating a beautiful future. I knew God was showing me that I had nothing to fear!

I was proud of myself and what I had created in a short year. I was growing fast and taking constant, massive actions toward my goals. I was a force to be reckoned with. I knew no one could stop me but me. So, I was unstoppable.

What have you let go of that led to opened doors?

We are all the same. We have dreams and goals, but sometimes we lose sight of what is important to us. We believe the lies that other people tell us about our abilities. However, the truth is that we are able to change. We are able to choose and decide to do things that bring us more joy and peace. We are all capable of focus and taking action steps no matter the circumstance we are living in. We are the creators of our own life, born with many talents and gifts. Creativity is our birthright. It doesn't matter where you are in life right now; you can still dream about your future. Decide what you desire and take action steps to make it happen.

Please accept the truth that you are the only one standing in your way by not doing what you need to do for yourself. People are going to say things to prevent you from reaching your potential. Oftentimes they have good intentions and are misguidedly saying things in an attempt to prevent you from failing. But that's not actually helpful. And even if you experience failures, you will learn from those failures and eventually succeed.

Please don't get me wrong, I know life is challenging. I have bad days. There are many times I feel like making excuses for why I can't change. I am tempted to do this because taking actions feels difficult.

For example, I was going through a challenging time in my life recently after I discovered that I was working with an unethical company. I knew I had to leave, but taking all the steps to quit and find a new job felt hard. For months, my soul was screaming loudly that I should get out, but the fear of not finding the right job and thinking everywhere was the same anyway, kept me there longer than I should have been.

And guess what, I started getting sick every few months. I rarely get ill. The only time I do is when I am stressed; my body shuts down and forces me to confront the problem, whether I want to or not.

While I was sick, I started watching a lot of TV. But then one day during my meditation, I was guided to cancel my cable TV. That was a rough thing to hear. I normally get the news on TV, and now, being unable to even sit up for long, TV was my only entertainment.

But I believed more in what I learned from meditation. I could not discount what my inner voice was telling me. I called my daughter and told her about my commitment to follow the voice of the spirit within. She was excited that I finally decided to cut out TV. She laughed at me gently and jokingly asked, "Mom, do you know there are other ways to be informed?"

That day I didn't watch TV at all to see how I would feel. At first, I felt I had lost something, but I pushed past that feeling, doing anything and everything else to keep myself busy. I even cleaned the house! The next day, I decided to cancel cable TV. Trust me when I tell you that I am not missing it at all. I have been able to work on my book and watch inspiring information on the internet. I am feeding my mind, and that makes me happy and content, bringing more peace into my life.

One week after cutting the television, I decided to let go of the job that was slowly killing me. I also decided not to look for another job. Instead, I kept working on myself, feeding what was right for my heart and spirit. My children thought their mother had gone crazy.

"Mom, maybe you can get your strength back and decide to look for another job later. Don't give up yet, Mom." They encouraged me to take care of myself fully, but also to remember there was hope. That was their way of saying they could count on me to do the right thing.

I remember my son came to visit me one day and noticed how happy and enthusiastic I was. He commented, "Mom, I am glad you are happy. I don't know what your plan is, but I know no matter what, you always manage to find your way and get back on your feet. You have done this for many years." It was his way to reassure me that he had faith in me.

I never thought my son had thought about me that way, but it sure gave me the courage and determination to find my way out of the darkness after a few weeks of hibernation. Knowing my family trusted me and had faith in my ability to make the right choice was the greatest gift they could have ever given me when nothing made sense. We are an exceptionally close family. We are involved in each other's lives and have always supported one another through difficult times. That's all we have. I learned what not to do or say to my children, from my family in Iran. As a result, I have taught my children well by my actions, and consequently, they are doing the same for me.

Love is the only thing that conquers all challenges. I believe in this statement with all my heart. Start loving yourself more each day. Start caring about your well-being every day. You are significant in spite of what others may have told you or believed about you. Your job is to be your own advocate and your own supporter even if no one else believes in you. I was in your shoes and know how it feels to be alone and scared to make any decisions. You have to start somewhere. What if you start today?

Begin by believing in your self-worth. Begin by believing in your gifts, talents, and dreams. There is a reason you have a dream – because deep within you, there is a power who knows you are capable of creating a life based on your needs and desires. Because you are worthy of having the best life like others do. Because you are good enough, smart enough and talented enough.

The key to creating a successful life is to decide what you genuinely want. Stop denying yourself from wanting to become a better version of yourself because you think it is unattainable. If you have difficulty finding what you want, start by analyzing your current situation and identify what you don't want.

What is currently in your life that is not serving you or making you happy? What are you not excited about? What's the boring and mundane life you are faced with day after day? Are you dreading going to work? Are you dreading going home to your family? Are you concerned about your health and well-being?

Knowing what you don't like about your current situation allows you to begin thinking about what you want to change. This can be a catalyst to help you discover what you want and where you wish to be. The rockets of desires begin flying when you stop resisting and allow yourself to receive the guidance. Your creativity and curiosity erupt like a volcano. The emotions that caused your pain and misery, will guide you to desire a better situation; a better partner, better job, better finances etc.

It's time to wake up and take control of your life. You are the master creator. You are the only one who has the power to make you happy. Not taking any chances based on fears and thoughts of not being good enough is detrimental to your livelihood. Don't waste any more time doing what makes you unhappy and miserable. You have only one life to live. Why don't you make this life count? What are you going to lose? There is no greater reward than finding your true self and your true worth. You do this by taking actions that will lead you to where you deserve to be.

The key to your success is in your capable hands. You are a powerful spirit who can move mountains if you want to. Try to make a decision today to do something that will improve your life. Perhaps you will decide to spend thirty minutes a day to become more informed on topics of interest to you. If you would like to see growth in your career, maybe you should research how to excel in your industry or improve your craft. If you desire to improve your interpersonal relationships, perhaps you should research effective methods of communication or how to heal from past hurts. Thirty minutes of research may not sound like enough time at first, but believe me, you will be happy you did. You will find the courage and motivation to continue to search for more answers. Likely, it will become a habit and you won't stop.

When I decided to take control of my life, I had no idea what was out there for me at all. I strongly suspect that you have more options than I had almost thirty years ago. I give you permission to be bold, to be fierce, and take action today. I am cheering you on, and holding you in my thoughts. Your future depends on the decision you make today!

Having difficulty making a decision? I am here to help.

www.soodabehmokry.com

info@soodabehmokry.com

Chapter Four

Step Three: The Importance of Mindset

We all have the potential to do and be anything we want. However, wanting something is not enough for us to achieve our goals. To an extent, doing something isn't even enough.

Our success is 20 percent based on our actions and skills, but 80 percent based on our mindset. We can go to school, learn new trends, and become licensed or certified in a special field, but without the right mindset, achieving goals becomes challenging.

What is Mindset?

Our mindset is our frame of mind. It's a set of attitudes, thoughts, beliefs, assumptions, notions, and feelings about our self-worth and ability to attain results in life. Our mindset is powerful. It impacts how we relate to others, and make sense of the world around us. It makes us believe we own certain qualities, intellectual aptitudes, talents, or gifts. Interestingly, our mindset forms early in our life. It is based on our perception of who we are which was shaped during childhood, before the age of six or seven.

Our mindset dictates our life. It determines what we focus on and how we view the world. Do we focus on abundance or on scarcity and lack? Do we move forward in life based on fear of failure, or do we take action because we desire success? Are we positive and view the world as a glass half-full? Or do we think negatively and critically and view the world as a glass half-empty?

A positive and strong mindset, which reinforces positive thoughts and beliefs about who we are, makes us move beyond fear and gives us the push we need to commit to pursuing our goals and dreams. We then decide to be accountable and take responsibility in our life. This enables us to create impact, become leaders, and succeed. Our thoughts and beliefs make up our mindset and our mindset plays a pivotal role in our life. Our thoughts and beliefs are significant in determining positive results in our journey. With the right mindset as our foundation, we discover strength and resilience. This leads us to success despite obstacles.

A negative mindset forces us to stay small, procrastinate, and never take action because we are mired in fear; we feel stuck in our path and eventually stop trying. This is an understandable thing. Our mind is designed to keep us safe, to alert us of dangerous situations. Its purpose is to protect us from an imminent life and death situation such as being faced by an angry animal or criminal. It tells us we can't cross a busy freeway due to the danger of being hit by a car. When our brain acts negatively, it is trying to protect us but, of course, it is really harming us.

Brain and Mindset

The brain is composed of two hemispheres: the left and the right. Some people function more left-brained while others are more right-brained. Whether one is left-brained or right-brained is determined by which side of the brain is most active. Those who are more artistic and creative tend to be right-brained. These people have great imaginations, intuition, and daydream more than their left-brained counterparts. They also tend to be more in tune with their feelings and emotions. The left-brainers among us are those who are more analytical, organized, and verbal.

Although these two hemispheres seem to function independently, they are connected by a bundle of nerves that communicate information constantly, so that the hemispheres work together as a complementary unit. Most people use the right side more than the left side or the left side more than the right, but we are all able to integrate the power of the brain to function better in life.

Our brain also has the power to constantly change and adapt. This allows the brain to create new habits and behavior. Although our brain is the command center of what we think, feel, and do, neuroscientists have discovered that our brain develops and transforms constantly. This is called *neuroplasticity*; the ability of the brain to change and reshape over time. The brain has the ability to form new pathways that allows the change to take place. As we learn and perform new tasks, new pathways actually develop, allowing us to form new habits. As we become disciplined in doing certain tasks, such as going to the gym daily, our brain becomes accustomed to doing so and creates a habit. Consequently, the action of going to the gym, which was difficult for a while, becomes a habit and easier to perform. We are constantly able to improve the quality of our life by training our brain to learn new skills.

All of that is amazing. Even if we are "left-brained", we can also use our right brain and our brain as a whole. Even if we've never gone to the gym, we can – and our brain will make that habit get easier over time. But here is something extra amazing, and of particular relevance to this chapter: the brain can't distinguish between what is real and what is imagined.

The brain responds to an imaginary situation as if we are actually physically experiencing it. That's the reason we actually sweat and tremble when we enter a dark room after hearing a mysterious sound. The intruder is imaginary, but our brain tells our body to react as though they are real. This is also why hypnosis has been successful in changing mindset and creating new neuro pathways that change behaviors. The brain uses the suggestions made by the hypnotherapist to create a new habit and discipline. In other words, when we change our perceptions, thoughts, and beliefs, the brain reacts and implements the information accordingly. This translates to new results.

How does perception and mindset affect our actions?

As I said, our mindset is established in childhood. An environment that allows children the freedom to express their thoughts and emotions leads them to be creative and resourceful in life. They become determined to focus on improving their lives, taking actions, and achieving results. They adapt a resilience mentality and learn to never give up. They discover there is no failure, but instead that they can embrace any results.

Or they can grow up in a restrictive, regressive environment. I grew up feeling not good enough. I believed I had no voice, that I had nothing important to say. I was unable to make any decision because I had learned I was not smart enough. I was unable to express myself because I had learned I had nothing worthy of saying. I believed these things because I'd been taught these things. Nothing about me seemed good enough for my mother.

Now, I know that she too was caught in a negative, weak mindset. She was unhappy. She was stuck in a life she didn't like. My father was barely around due to the nature of his job, and we lived far from my mother's family because of my father's work. So, she had almost no help raising us children, and she had her own full-time job outside the home. Exhausted from a long day at work, she would angrily yell at us if we were having fun and playing. "You will end up crying if you laugh too much."

At the time, this sounded like nonsense. I'd hiccupped from laughing too hard, but how would laughter lead to crying? But as if she had created a self-fulfilling prophecy, we kids inevitably would start quarreling, and then she got to say, "See, I told you someone was going to cry!" Eventually, I made sense of all this as a fact that I was not supposed to be happy. Every time life was good,

I would wonder when the other shoe was going to drop. I would fear what was coming next. Believing it made it real for me.

I had no other role model to show me anything different, so I moved on in life believing everything my mother had said. I felt stupid because, instead of telling me I was as smart as anyone else and had the potential to do better, my mother would make me feel lesser than.

"Why can't you get an A+, Soodabeh?" she would say. "Do you think those who always get good grades have more than two eyes? Do they have a better life than you? No, they just work harder. Why can't you do the same?" She would continue expressing her thoughts, "I work hard. I provide a roof over your head. The only thing I am asking you to do is to study. Is that too much to ask?"

I also felt invisible because no one ever told me anything other than that I was short. "Maybe we can get you some hormone shots. They say that works," Mom had suggested more than once. Then she learned that might not be effective. "Well, I heard it may affect more than just your height," she said one day. "I am afraid trying to get you taller may make one leg grow longer than the other."

I was numb, just listened to what new thing she would come up with every day. I didn't feel important enough to say anything even when decisions were being made on my behalf.

I lived with these thoughts and beliefs of inadequacy until I moved to America and was abandoned by my husband. Life forced me to do something about my belief system, I guess. I am not sure why things happen the way they do. I have no answers, to be honest. It took me a lot of heartache and struggle to find out who I really was. At first, anger, and resentment toward my mother came to surface. Why had she treated me that way? Why did she hate me so much?

Then I learned the truth. I was a constant reminder of my mother's unsatisfied life. Her broken dreams. Her unhappy and unfulfilled marriage. She was reacting to her own negative mindset.

She really wanted a better life for me. I believe that with all my heart, even if it doesn't make sense to you now. I learned to forgive her and have compassion for her because she taught me what not to do. She taught me to be a better mother than her. She taught me not to give up on my dreams like she did, or like she felt she had to.

Now, I can remember my mother's hard work and dedication to provide a better life for her children. I know she loved us dearly. She never intended to hurt us. But she didn't have a positive role model growing up either. No one taught her how to behave, communicate, work or care for her children and household by herself.

I learned compassion for my mother when life put me in a place to understand her sufferings. I cried for her, and I cried for my grandmothers, and I cried for every single woman who came before me. I still feel their pain and struggles. As I write this, I feel emotional, and tears flow on my face.

The patriarchal society, in both Iran and in the United States, has silenced women for generations. Society ranks us as inferior regardless of where we live in the world. We have to cook and clean, work outside the home to provide for our family, raise our children and be good parents. Where is the mutual law, or morality clause that dictates this as a fact?

Trust me, I am not against men. I feel compassion for men who have also suffered in silence because society expects them to be strong and to tolerate everything without any complaints. I want to reach out and tell men they are good enough even though they feel inadequate at times because they too were told they weren't good enough. That's the reason for violent behavior. That's the main reason men attack women. They are told to hold their anger and frustration in. No wonder they explode like volcanoes.

My dear friends, I know your pain. I have been in your shoes. I know the struggles of trying to keep your head up and pretend that everything is okay. You feel stuck and like you have nowhere to go. You can't sleep at night because you are not sure what will happen tomorrow. You are scared- you live in a state of constant fear and anxiety. You need help. You need support. You have paid for many programs without results.

I have done it all too. I have spent money buying from infomercials: tapes, DVD's, CDs, and many programs. I searched and searched for something to ease my pain. I collected many workout videos and pieces of exercise equipment over the years, each time stopping that specific exercise regimen after only a week or two. Then they were moved to the garage to make room for the new ones. Nothing eased my pain until I learned to work on my mindset and feelings of unworthiness.

Hopeless and Stuck

Working on our mindset should be our number one priority before taking action. If we don't, we may feel resistance, make excuses, and start procrastinating what is required to get to the next step.

Sometimes we are not even aware of our self-sabotage because it's coming from really deep in the subconscious mind. Fear appears when we are trying to do something different, to change, and to create something new. You may sabotage a great relationship because, deep inside, you don't believe you are good enough or worthy of being loved. You may take one step forward and a few steps back, or go around in a circle, and never accomplish what you have started. Trust me, I have done all of this because my subconscious believed the lies I was told about my worth growing up. I procrastinated on projects. I would stop what I was doing to start something new; then I would move on to the next project before finishing that task. I was running in a circle chasing my tail! I was in a cage, running on a hamster wheel.

I am also speaking from what I have seen working with many clients for the past twenty years. We are all the same in that we have the same type of brain. The reason why some people succeed in life, business, or relationships and some don't is the direct result of our mindset and what we believe about ourselves.

I have noticed some people blame others for their lack of success. They blame their parents, teachers, and the environment they grew up in. I agree that our past experiences play an important role in the condition of our life but refusing to find a solution to our challenges is not a productive way to live. There is no accountability and responsibility when we use the blame game and choose the victim mentality.

In my practice as a nurse and a hypnotherapist, I have observed that some people would rather focus on anger, resentment, and blame because they know if they let these feelings go, they have to do something about their lives. One of my clients (I'll call her Jenny for the sake of this story) never wanted to let go of the past. She was stuck, but unwilling to do anything about it.

"I don't want to forgive my mother, ever!" she cried. Her face was red with tears washing over her face. "She ruined my life. She criticized me until the day she died. I hate her. It's because of her that I can't have a good relationship. I can't feel good about myself. I can't lose weight. I can't believe you are asking me to forgive her, Soodabeh."

She went on and on convincing me why she had to remain angry. "But Jenny, you know she is gone and has no control over you. The power is within your capable hands. You can decide right now to let go of the past and drop the heavy baggage you have carried for many years, dear one. You don't need to feel this way anymore." I persuaded her every time she came to visit me. She wanted a magical remedy to feel better; to be more successful in her relationships, but no one can carry shame, guilt, and anger yet expect a peaceful life.

Jenny's mindset had set her up for failure. She believed what she was told by her mother. Jenny had chosen that way of life for herself by refusing to change her mindset. She had many choices in life. She could have stopped hurting by trying to learn to love herself; to say goodbye to the lies she heard growing up from her mother and other family members. The sad thing is that she chose not to. She was in control of her feelings and emotions and chose to hold on to the thoughts of being a victim rather than allowing love and victory to come into her experiences.

The point of this story is to show you that refusing to let go of hurt feelings and errors in thinking will hinder your success. You must choose to no longer accept the lies that you have been told. Instead, aspire towards a different and better mindset. We can't go through life holding onto our past negative experiences and expect to see love, joy, and positive encounters in our reality. It's not possible. Even if you grew up believing that you weren't good enough, there are ways to overcome any residual feelings of self-doubt, and thoughts of unworthiness. We have the power to focus on negativity or try to learn how to let go, forgive, and move on.

I have noticed that some people- men and women- tend to stay in an unfulfilled relationship and commit adultery for years. Jenny did the same. She didn't love herself but wanted to find a man who would love her unconditionally. She would put herself in a situation with married men and expected them to be kind and loving toward her. It was impossible for her to find anything but disaster.

I am not trying to judge people for having a different lifestyle. What I am trying to say is that, unless we are ready to let what is not serving us go, we won't find something better. The limited mindset holds us hostage if we don't change. We become a prisoner of life without our control or efforts. When we find ourselves living an unfulfilled life, we need to focus our attention on finding solutions that work. Something must change before we can live a more enriching and satisfying life.

How Changing My Mindset Changed My Life Trajectory

Surviving nursing school was one of the hardest experiences of my life. I was faced with an instructor who was prejudiced. She believed only young, white people had the right to attend nursing school. She would create issues for every student who was over the age of thirty, or who was a person of color. She even forced several students to give up and drop out of the program. So, she obviously didn't like me and believed I should not be allowed to attend the program.

This was particularly shocking to me because until then, in my little world, I hadn't experienced racism. Growing up I learned to accept everyone, and everyone seemed to be accepted. To me, going to school in a diverse environment wasn't a surprise or something I had to struggle with. I saw the majority of people as trying to help me, and only 1 percent of people weren't. Suddenly, I was faced with that 1 percent.

The feeling of being persecuted by my teacher brought back old fears and memories of being tortured in Iran. I worked constantly to learn to be fluent in English while completing my assignments. I had been a nurse for ten years in Iran, and believed I was perfect for the program because of my background. I was fluent in medical terminology because we used Latin terminology in Iran; the same terminology used in the medical world in America.

I frequently had thoughts that I was not good enough and not worthy enough. *Maybe she is right, maybe I am not supposed to be a part of the program. Maybe I should stop.*

But then, I had nothing without going to school and trying to create a better life for my family. I decided to talk with my advisor, Linda, one day to seek solutions.

"Soodabeh, we have a department of affirmative action here. Make an appointment and go to see them for advice. They know how to handle the situation legally and appropriately. You have nothing to worry about. "

The next day, I went to talk with Mark, at the affirmative action department in my college. He listened to what I had to say and after looking at my grades which were all A or B, Mark leaned back in his chair and smiled. "Soodabeh, you haven't done anything wrong. You have been working hard as your grades are showing us. You speak fluent enough for me or anyone to understand. You are eligible to continue the program." Mark shook my hand and escorted me to the door.

Although I felt relieved to know I was fortunate enough to have the protections of those in the right place taking my side and allowing me to continue the program, I realized this might be the beginning of a difficult life living in America. I was filled with fears, self-doubt, and uncertainties. This experience had already affected me in the deepest level of my subconscious possible.

What if I can't succeed? What if everyone is right and I am not good enough to complete the program?

Our challenges are blessings sometimes. I was faced to look at the deepest part of my psyche and try to correct it. I was faced to deal with a mindset of unworthiness and the subconscious blocks that kept coming to surface to be healed. Facing and dealing with these issues as they surfaced allowed me to become whole again. This complete healing allowed me to appreciate the events of my past because they prepared me for my future. Facing all the challenges growing up with a strict mother, was the blessing I needed to survive the challenges I was facing while attending nursing school.

Experiencing the challenge of dealing with my nursing advisor and the subconscious mind regarding my worthiness had made me afraid to go to school. The fears had come to surface to the point where I was scared to take tests, because I believed I would fail.

"I can't believe she is doing this. This is the only chance I have to make a good life for my family. What am I going to do now? I can't quit, but I am afraid I will fail." I was crying and trying to explain my situation to Linda.

"Soodabeh, I suggest you go to see one of the advisors who is trained in techniques to help you succeed."

I left her office and went straight to talk to Natasha, one of the college advisors. She was sitting, looking down at a book on her lap. Her curly, dark blond hair shielded her face. She stood up when I said hello, her light gray pantsuit smoothing into place, and she offered her hand.

Natasha listened attentively to my concerns, and after I was finished, she smiled and said, "I know how to help you. Have you heard anything about guided imagery or visualization techniques?"

"No, I haven't."

"Well, I guess you are going to learn today. Are you willing to try it with me?" She said with a sweet smile showing her pearly white teeth.

It was the first time someone had intervened to give me a tool I was going to utilize for the rest of my life. I was willing to do anything. I had no idea what guided imagery was, but I decided to give it a try if doing the exercise could help me pass my classes.

"Close your eyes and take a deep breath," she said softly. Now imagine you are in the most beautiful place you have ever been. Take deep breaths and exhale. As you breathe in, inhale peace and calm, and as you exhale, let go of all your fears and anxiety." She continued.

Natasha gradually helped me to go deeper and deeper to become completely relaxed. "Now, imagine you are in your class, sitting on the chair and taking the test. What do you see? What do you hear? How does the chair feel?" she continued. "Now, I want you to take a deep breath as you look at questions, one after another. Feel your body filled with relaxation and peace. Take another deep breath and imagine you know all the answers." She continued asking me to take deep breaths again.

"Now, I want you to imagine you are outside the office, right by the big glass window. You are going to see the results of the tests posted on the glass window. What do you see, Soodabeh?" she instructed me to take more deep breaths. "Now you can feel relaxed and in peace seeing your name on the white paper on the window. You have passed your test!"

That was the way we knew if we had passed tests. The names of whom had passed the tests would be on a paper taped inside of the glass window. Being able to visualize the same process I would have seen later on, became ingrained in my mind's eyes for a better result.

At first, I had no idea if guided imagery would help me, but as I worked with Natasha each week, I felt more relaxed and at ease. I felt a confidence I had never had before. I began remembering her words even when I wasn't working with her. She had changed my fear and anxiety of test taking to strength and confidence. Twenty to thirty minutes, and a few times a week had worked magic, and I was able to pass my tests and go to the next level.

Change Your Mind, Change Your Circumstance

One of my own experiences to share occurred a few years ago when I had just moved back to Portland and was working as a home health nurse. It was a good working environment until the management changed. The one who took the position didn't like me. Mike had never worked directly with patients as a nurse, but worked as an educator in the office. Consequently, he had no clue what others were doing working directly with patients.

Mike kept finding issues about what I had said and the way I worked while taking care of my patients. He spent countless hours keeping a log of my work hours. Looking from 8:00 am to 5:00 pm only, he discovered that I never worked past 2:00 or 3:00 pm. Working in a home health setting, I had flexible hours. As long as I completed my assignments and kept a log of my hours, I was in compliance with the expectations of my job.

I would start in the morning and log in, check my emails, work on documentation, call the doctors, and then go to visit patients. We had the option of not charting at the patient's home because it was distracting; constantly staring at the computer didn't allow us to be fully present and attentive to the patient's needs. So, I would go home, rest, relax, eat, and start working to complete my documentation after 5:00 pm.

If Mike would have reached out and asked me the rationale rather than jumping to conclusion, I would have told him the reason why my time log was reflecting that I clocked out at 2:00 pm. If he would have run the log until 10:00 pm every evening, he would have noticed I was working long hours every day. Mike's limited mindset and thoughts of who I was, caused him to make the wrong decision based on false assumption. Instead of giving me a chance, he decided to make the mistake of accusing me of cheating.

One day, my director, Susan, called and asked me to go have a meeting with her. I had already known the other manager, Mike, didn't like me for whatever reason. I had already experienced him creating challenges for me by changing my schedule and giving my patients to another nurse. I went to the office and saw Mike, Susan, and Mary, the other manager who trained me when I started working there, all sitting across the table. My intuition was telling me it wasn't going to be good news since I was sitting on the other side of them.

"Soodabeh, you are here because we have noticed that you go home after 2:00 pm every day but lead us to believe you are working longer hours by asking for overtime sometimes. We are not accepting of this kind of behavior. I have kept a log of your time and have to write you up today."

I let Mike explain everything he had to say. I had tears in my eyes thinking about my past experiences of dealing with those who have accused me of things I had never done based on their lack of clarity and narrow mindset. I already knew Mike didn't like me. But what was hurting me at that moment, was to see both Susan and Mary sitting there and not protecting me. I had a great work relationship with Susan since she was the one who interviewed me when I was in California. I had a good work relationship with Mary because she trained me and had already seen how I work with my patients. I felt betrayed by those I trusted.

"Mike, you are wrong for accusing me of things I have never done. I am an ethical and hardworking individual and care about what I do. I have never been treated with so much disrespect since the day you started working as my manager. You have no idea what it takes to work with patients every day. If you would have asked me the first time you saw this issue, I would have explained the situation. But you didn't respect me enough to give me a chance. Instead, you assumed I was a bad person." I expressed my thoughts firmly and tried so hard to prevent tears from falling down.

"Working with patients doesn't mean that we have to complete our documentation while at the patient's home. I go home and start again after taking a break because I don't have time to take a break earlier during the day. I finish visiting my patients and complete my documentations later. This is the way I have always been working and no one had any issues with this. If you would have checked the log into the evening hours, you would have seen how late I work every night."

At this time, I noticed everyone was quiet. Susan's face was pale, staring at the floor at this point. Mary's face red with frowning while looking at Mike. Neither one of them were looking directly at me. I explained my side of the story about how I had constantly been harassed by Mike and never said anything. I saw Mary and Susan's jaw dropped as I kept explaining the incidents.

I was a new employee there and had been working for less than five months. I was fearful of losing my job and not being able to pay the bills. My fears and the mindset of not good enough had allowed me to tolerate Mike for a few months. I thought maybe he would eventually change. I expected someone else to change his behavior for me. It was wrong. I should have known that it was not going to happen, but I feared losing my job.

I had to make a decision and choose to either continue working in a toxic environment with people who questioned my integrity and work ethic until I found another job, or just leave. I cried all day in my car and between visits with my patients. I was scared that, if I left the company, I wouldn't be able to find a job I wanted. More importantly, I knew that staying in a hostile work environment would be toxic for me. I emailed my resignation just a few hours later.

Susan approached me and begged me to stay, "Please Soodabeh. I know you. I hired you. I love you. I have faith in you and what you have done for the past few months. Please don't leave." She knew she would lose a great and hardworking nurse.

"I respect myself too much to put up with someone who questions my integrity without the willingness to at least communicate their concerns. I am afraid I have to go."

Working on my mindset for many years, and discovering my self-worth, I knew I deserved better. I chose to leave no matter what Susan, or anyone would say or offer. I had accepted this job while working in California and trying to move back to Portland quickly. I accepted the position knowing that it paid much less than I was worthy of receiving due to fear of not finding a better job. The challenge I was facing at that time was a blessing in fact. I was able to find another job that paid much more than the job I left, and my bosses and coworkers respected me far more than the people who worked at my previous place of employment.

I have many stories that display the benefits that I have received from living life with a healthy mindset. I didn't always live like that. I stayed in destructive relationships because I didn't know how to love myself. I was seeking approval from someone else acknowledging my existence. I allowed others to abuse me, verbally and emotionally, because of the fear of being alone for the rest of my life. I wasn't aware of the issues at first because it was deep within my subconscious. I kept complaining about the fact that I was unable to attract a loving man in my life rather than trying to change myself first.

For many years, like many women I wanted a hero to come and rescue me. I thought that, because I had endured many challenges, I deserved a savior. I was unaware of the lack of self-worth deep within me. Instead of trying to find solace in myself, I was searching for approval from others. I was waiting for them to prove that I was worthy and deserving of being loved.

"No one loves me!" I used to say this statement for years. It took me a long time to realize I was wrong. I was surrounded by many people- family, friends, my patients- who loved and adored me beyond my limited belief. But I chose to believe otherwise because I didn't have a romantic partner to acknowledge me.

Every time I felt blocked by an invisible wall of disapproval, I became more doubtful of my self-worth. I remembered my mother telling me we weren't lucky. She believed we were doomed to have less. We were meant to be miserable. Suffering was our motto. I accepted the lies that she was told by her family while growing up. Lies that said she was condemned to a life of misery. She was never able to be happy, always focused on the pain of the past or concerned about the future. She was unable to find a good man to love her after my father died. I, eventually, felt I inherited the bad luck and was doomed to suffer for the rest of my life.

I remember working with one of my mentors, Bryan, about the subject of love and romantic relationships. Bryan looked at me and said, "when you are ready to be loved and in a good relationship, you will find the right man willing to love you just the way you are. However, you need to start loving yourself first. You need to accept you are worthy and deserving."

Although I never said anything to him physically due to respect, I was upset with him for a very long time. *How dare he tell me that! I know I deserve better. Haven't I gone through enough? When do I deserve to have a man to love and comfort me?*

Many years later and after learning about the power of mindset, everything made sense to me as I learned to love and respect myself. I don't claim to be perfect, but I try to be the best version of myself daily. I do this because I believe I am worthy and deserving of happiness. I don't need others to tell me I am good or beautiful or even worthy of certain experiences. I know I am worthy, and that makes me happy and content. I am at peace everyday knowing that I am truly valuable. It is because of this knowledge that I no longer feel the need to seek outside approval. This is the power of a healthy mindset. I know I am enough!

Food for Thought

You, my dear friends, are also enough. You matter. You are brilliant. You are magnificent. You are creative. You have the power to be or do whatever you desire. Don't you ever dare give up on yourself. Work on your mindset every day and see the magic as you change.

If you are determined to change your circumstances, you need to start by discovering what is going on inside of you. What do you think of yourself? What do you think about your self-worth? Do you love and respect yourself, or do you allow others to treat you like a doormat? Are you assertive and willing to let people know what is on your mind, or do you expect others to read your mind and get upset when they don't? Focus and see what situations and circumstances in your everyday life make you unhappy. Knowing what you don't want, guides you to search for something better. It also allows you to have more meaningful experiences in life.

The struggle is real. What we know in the back of our mind about who we are is real to us. Although it is not accurate. We learned it over the years growing up. We believed in lies our parents and teachers, and family and friends told us. They made us believe we are not good enough. I will repeat this over and over again for you to understand the following key piece of information:

The only thing that can stop you from reaching your full potential is what YOU feel and believe about yourself.

I want to help you. I want you to know that you are capable of creating the life you desire. I want to hold your hands and look into your eyes and say you are good enough. You matter. You are significant. You are strong, and you are brilliant. I hope the stories I share in this book will resonate with you and motivate you to take positive action in your life. I hope the stories will encourage you to abandon the error in thinking that you are incapable of producing positive results in life and replace it with knowledge, courage, and strength.

Life happens outside of our control. We all face challenges. But we all have the ability to decide to do something to change our outcomes. We are always in control of our life. We have the strength to do and be what we desire in spite of our obstacles.

We all have some degree of self-doubt. Those who succeed in life, are the ones who push beyond fears and negative chatter in the mind. I have learned to redirect my negative self-talk every day. It never ends; you just learn to master it.

Every time you achieve a goal, remind yourself you can do more and become more. Success is not a sprint. It's about taking massive actions every single day. In the next chapter, I offer some techniques for getting there.

Chapter Five
Tools for Daily Mindset Work

I have many stories about the power of mindset. Every struggle and challenge I have experienced in life brought me closer to accepting and understanding the powerful spirit that lives within me. I discovered my strengths, and mastered the art of self-love. Now, I embrace life challenges and try to learn the lesson in every situation. When we fight life challenges instead of allowing them to make us better, we become enslaved by our circumstances. Remaining teachable allows us to grow and makes us more equipped to deal with our circumstances. It is through surrender that we gain victory.

Learning and accepting these facts allowed me to replace anger, pain, and suffering with healing, forgiveness, and compassion for myself and others. Once I realized that every experience is here to teach me something, it became easier for me to let go of attitudes and beliefs that didn't serve me. By changing my mindset, my thoughts, and my beliefs, I have been able to create more joyful experiences and become more successful in life. For me, success is not having more material possessions, but having more peace, greater joy, and the knowledge that all is well in my world in the face of all challenges. That's the true meaning of success.

Being a certified hypnotherapist and NLP practitioner, I am always helping others with their mindset. I am good at my job because I have experienced these issues in my personal life.

I teach my clients what I taught myself; how to be conscious of our thoughts every day. I have discovered many tools over the years that have helped me and my clients to do this. You may connect with one tool or try to implement all of the tools you learn in this chapter.

One important fact that you need to remember is that there are no magic remedies. Consistency is key. People often make the mistake of practicing a few days or weeks and then they stop practicing because they assume they have mastered it all. Doing this is like going to the gym for a few weeks and expecting that effort to last your entire lifetime. It simply does NOT work that way. Maintaining a positive mindset is a daily practice. I devote time to practicing the tools that work for me every single day – yes every day – because I want to see results.

The Power of Meditation

Have you ever woken up and felt immediately that it would be a bad day? You have no idea why, but it feels like everything will go the wrong way no matter what you do. Well, you are not alone. I had these experiences until I learned about the power of meditation.

As soon as I wake up, my mind is running nonstop. So, I decided to calm it by engaging it in meditation. As I was searching for a way to quiet my mind and master the art of meditation, I realized that focusing on simple gratitude techniques allows my mind to be active which is it's preferred state. It also seems to retrain it to focus on the positive, rather than the negative.

For example, I usually wake up feeling anxious so I began my day by trying to focus on my immediate surroundings; where I am in my bed, what is around me etc. I then focus on being grateful for what I have at that moment, such as a comfortable bed, the warmth of my blanket, the comfort of my pillow etc.

I typically spend ten to fifteen minutes resting in this place of gratitude and focusing on what I am feeling at that moment. This is called *active meditation.* In active meditation you ask your mind to participate rather than becoming quiet. When we ask our mind to focus, it will respond immediately. Begin from a place of cooperation with your mind.

I noticed that, when I practiced this every morning before getting out of bed, I would have pleasant days. I would experience less challenges, less stress and I even found myself dealing with difficult people less frequently. The truth is that focusing on gratitude allows our mind to be set and primed for the day. The first thing I was doing every day was asking my mind to search for positive experiences. That way, later in the day, if something appeared challenging, I would be able to find a solution without feeling out of control and stressed out. My mind was pre focused on positive experiences.

Gradually, I was able to meditate later in the evening and then before going to bed. I would start by focusing on the positive experiences I wanted to create the next day. I would express thanks for all the blessings I had observed throughout that day. The more I focused on positive experiences, the more I attracted them. It was magical. I was the creator of my life. I was in total control and able to act and respond to situations in a positive manner.

I still have difficulty quieting my mind completely, but I am always able to use the power of active meditation to my advantage. That's a gift. Even though I am not able to completely quiet my creative, questioning mind, I am able to guide it by being aware of my thoughts and feelings.

In other words, I am always trying to be conscious of everything that is happening inside of me, which gives me the tools to act based on facts when facing a challenging situation rather than reacting based on anger and fear. This takes us to the next tool I would like to share with you.

Working with the Divine Source and Spirit

Those who have read my first book, *Angel Nightingale*, know I am a spiritual person. I learned the power of working with the spirit and the angelic realm many years ago when I was very depressed and trying to make sense of my previous challenges and the challenges I was facing at the time. What I learned then was to allow God, the Divine Source, the Universe, and the power of the angelic realm to help me.

For me, believing in a power greater than my physical body has allowed me to face every challenge with grace and dignity. I am not trying to preach a certain belief, but to inform you of what has worked for me. Operating with an awareness of the spiritual realm has allowed me to be happier and full of life. It's not about being religious, but knowing we are not alone. It's about having faith that, no matter how we feel, there is always a solution to the challenges we face. This mindset alone is empowering.

Connecting with God, angels, and the Divine Source has allowed me to know I am always protected. I have a powerful group of invisible friends and guides helping me every step of the way. Connecting with this powerful source every morning before my gratitude meditation has allowed me to feel more comfortable and at ease regarding what is ahead of me. I also have been able to use the power of the Source to help my clients and my patients every day for the past twenty years. Knowing and believing in something greater than my physical body has allowed me to feel peace of mind rather than letting fear creep in. I share more information and stories about this topic in my first book, *Angel Nightingale*. In the meantime, if you have any questions, you can simply send me an email at <u>info@soodabehmokry.com</u>. I will be more than happy to assist you.

The Art of Journaling

I love to write. It helps me to know where I am in life. It allows me to analyze my situation and seek for answers. I have always encouraged clients to start writing. Your journal is not like a diary you used to have when you were a teenager, for example. It's serious business. It's about you and the power that helps and guides you to get to know yourself better. You are not trying to write a book for others. No one is going to judge you. It's one of the most effective ways to be aware of what is going on inside your mind. Journaling reveals insights about what is within you. It reveals the most intimate thoughts and beliefs you were never aware of.

To make journaling easier, begin by sitting in a comfortable place and start by focusing on gratitude. Watch your thought patterns about what you believe regarding your life. Do you feel you can easily write about the topic of gratitude every day, or are you having difficulty doing so? Is your glass half-full or half-empty? Don't judge what comes to the surface. Maybe you are experiencing a challenging life situation and don't know what will happen to you tomorrow. Maybe you are fearful of where you are in life and have no way to look at what is working at the moment.

We can't always be happy and in an uplifting mood. It's not normal to always be cheerful. I know because I have been in your shoes before. I am not going to preach and expect you to always be happy. However, I want to provide tools you can utilize even in the most challenging of times, so that you can identify small things that make you appreciate life. Focusing on the positive will train your mind to recognize even more positive situations and experiences throughout the day. If you expect great things to happen, you will prove yourself right! Ask and you shall receive! Seek and you shall find!

For example, being a nurse and witnessing people being seriously ill, losing their independence and their ability to eat, sit, walk, or even talk, has helped me to be grateful for these basic abilities. I am alive, I can talk, I can walk. I can eat, drink and feel. Most of us have heard the common phrase "Don't take things for granted!" After hearing it so often, it can sound cliché but it is said so often because it is a sound piece of advice; a forewarning that people should live with gratitude or else they could live to regret it.

So, if you are in the worst position in your life, consider the fact that you are alive. Consider your ability to talk, feel, see, and hear. Start there and the rest will reveal itself as you focus and train your mind to look for positive experiences.

You may have a dream you don't feel comfortable sharing with your friends and family. Writing will allow you to express your feelings and emotions. Start writing your feelings and thoughts, both positive and negative, in your notebook or journal. This allows you to see them physically and feel the words as they are coming out of your mind before being captured on the paper.

See how you feel as you write them or think about them. What is the message? Does thinking about your dream make you fearful? Does it make you feel alive? Nervous? Intimidated? Are your thoughts trying to make you aware of any dangers you might be facing? One of the biggest secrets journaling can uncover is how your own mind might be sabotaging you. It also brings hidden thoughts and concerns to the surface so you can face these issues head on. For most people, seeing a dream on paper makes it more real to them. We can write about a number of different things. Try writing about what is in the forefront of your mind. If you write long enough without distractions and really focus on writing what is on your mind, eventually your deepest thoughts and feelings will surface. It's your job to put them on paper!

If you are trying to change your life for the better – for example, you may want to go back to school or get out of a go-nowhere relationship – you may notice your mind trying to convince you of reasons why you shouldn't do what you want. Journaling can help you investigate these feelings more thoroughly and find solutions .

Maybe you were told you weren't a good student in the past by your family or teachers. Now, you are in a situation that requires you to go back to school to obtain certain certifications or even a diploma. You have been working long hours at your current job, taking care of your family, and now you have to make a decision to find time in your busy schedule to go back to school for more training.

What does your mind say when you are trying to make this difficult decision? In order to keep you safe, so that what happened in the past concerning education doesn't happen again, your mind might look for excuses why you don't have time to pursue your dreams.

You are unaware of this truth at first. You don't realize that your mind remembers the pain you previously experienced while going to school. You thought you were healed as you grew up.

Our minds remember things vividly even though we consciously don't remember them. So, writing in a journal allows your subconscious to become more proactive in searching for solutions. Be frank and ask direct questions as if you are trying to have a conversation with a friend. Your mind may produce answers to the questions or it might just use the questions as a starting point to generate additional thoughts, ideas and hidden feelings. When we write, more than just thinking is activated. We can physically see the problem, which allows us to analyze and understand what has been written.

When I decided to write my first book, *Angel Nightingale*, I had to go deep within to remember what had happened. I had to be willing to remember unpleasant and terrifying events I had put to rest for decades. But as I began writing, more and more information came to the surface. At times, remembering the details of each event became impossible and unbearable, but

I knew I had a purpose. I took a break sometimes, but then I pushed through the feelings of grief as I remembered my dark past. I knew I was in a better place and not directly at the event. That's the power we have; we can remind ourselves we are not stuck in the past, and we are safe in the present moment.

As you learn to write your feelings and emotions, you will become more conscious of what is in your mind. You will learn the root of all of your issues. Knowing why you act a certain way or do things differently than others helps you to make better choices in your life. You become more aware of what you feel and why you feel a certain way. You will understand, for example, the reason why you were so bothered by something someone said. It probably wasn't what they said exactly – but what event from your past that your mind remembered and connected to what they said.

Trust me, I know this feeling very well. I perceived I wasn't a good student because my mother always expected me to be better. I took her constant expectations of me working harder as my weakness; I felt I was not smart enough to get better grades. Many years later when I had to go back to school in America, my fears blocked me at first but, as I worked harder, studied every day and got good results, I became more confident in myself and my ability to be successful in school.

I noticed this with work too. I strived for years to understand why I was attracting the same kind of managers over and over. I was trying hard to be the perfect employee, yet I always felt they were judging me and telling me I wasn't good enough.

Expressing my emotions in my journal one day, I discovered the truth when I wrote, "She reminds me of my mother!" I was shocked. At that moment, I realized that I had been trying to make my mother happy for years without success. No matter what I did, I always seemed to fall short. I carried this sense of inadequacy into adulthood so I was operating from a place of unworthiness. That is why I felt like my performance was never good enough despite going above and beyond to overperform. Deep down inside, I believed I was inadequate so I assumed that my bosses felt the same way about me. As a result, I was overly sensitive to criticism.

Then came a sigh of relief. With that knowledge, I felt the chains were broken and I was free at last. It feels great to feel the freedom from the limited thoughts your mind makes you believe day after day. I no longer feel like my bosses are displeased and judging me. Why? Because I chose to disassociate from the lie that I am inadequate and that nothing I do will ever be good enough.

Once I realized the truth that was buried deep within my psyche, I became more powerful than ever before. I was able to approach my manager and ask for a raise even though the company was in the middle of a transition and laying people off. That's the honest truth. I was no longer working from a place of unworthiness. Instead, I chose to embrace the truth which is that I am worthy and deserving of being recognized for my hard work. I accepted my worth rather than expecting others to do it for me. With this new found sense of self-worth, I felt bold and capable so I requested a pay raise.

No one would have acknowledged or offered to give me a raise had I not been bold enough to ask for one. And I could have never done that without first understanding where my negative mindset came from. Journaling helped me do that.

The Power of Creative Visualization

Another useful tool to change your mindset is to visualize what you want to accomplish. I learned this technique from my advisor, Natasha, when I was having difficulty in nursing school. (I shared it in the previous chapter)

As my children became teenagers, they preferred to spend time with their friends rather than be with me. I felt vulnerable and concerned that my children didn't need me any longer because they were so independent. I had worked very hard to create a better life for my family and it felt like I was being cheated out of precious time with them. Consequently, I had no family to be with. I began grieving this loss and started questioning my purpose.

My inquisitive mind wanted to know who I was and where I came from. I believe that being aware of these questions led me to notice a TV program talking about the power of creative visualization. I bought a book on the subject and began to practice what I had learned. It was amazing and fulfilling knowing I had the power to be anywhere I wanted to by just imagining the place I desired to be. It became joyful to be at home sitting on the sofa and trying to visualize life on the beach.

Some people don't believe in the power of mind and imagination. So, if you are one of them, let's try this exercise. Close your eyes and imagine you are in a beautiful garden full of lemon trees. Just the thought of lemons makes my mouth water as I am trying to write. Now imagine you are reaching with your hand and picking up a plump lemon. Can you feel and smell the fresh lemon? Now, picture yourself taking it to your kitchen and pick up a knife then cut the lemon in half. How do you feel now? What senses are erupting in pleasure?

That is the power of imagination. Our mind doesn't understand or differentiate an experience from imagination. You feel as if you are physically squeezing the lemon juice in your mouth. Do you get the point?

You may have heard of the Reticular Activating System (RAS). It's a network of neurons located in the brain stem that notices things when we focus on them. For example, when you buy a new red car, you began noticing more red cars as you drive every day. This is the direct result of activating your RAS.

When we are imagining, we activate the RAS as if we have already experienced certain events.

You can use the power of imagination to make a difference in the outcome of your desires. When you are clear on what you want, use the power of creative visualization as a tool to see, feel, sense, and create the experience and outcome in your mind. Your body and mind create a sense of certainty to the point where you begin feeling it in your heart. Visualization activates RAS and produces magnificent results.

Imagine and focus on what you want to create as if it has already been done. Immerse yourself in the positive emotions and feelings of accomplishment as you witness the result. If you want to go to school, but are afraid of the outcome, start by imagining your end result. Picture yourself in your mind's eyes wearing a cap and gown on the stage to receive your degree. You are born with tools to create anything you wish and dreamed of. Use these tools to your advantage and stop trying to make excuses for why you are not good enough to do something you have yearned to do for years.

The Beauty of Mirror Work

Another tool is what Louise Hay has taught in her books for many years, called mirror work. You begin by looking at yourself in the mirror and expressing words of love and positivity to influence better confidence and self-esteem. I remember the first time I stood in my bathroom in front of the mirror, trying to tell myself I was beautiful. I had such a difficult time voicing this statement to the point where I couldn't even look at myself. I was also shocked that I hadn't realized how I had felt about myself till then. It was sad for me to acknowledge that I was unable to say such a simple statement to myself.

Looking back at that moment many years ago and writing these words is making me emotional even now. I remember a small, dark face staring at herself in the mirror, shocked and in awe by the realization that had just taken place.

Although it was very difficult for me to say I was beautiful, I didn't give up trying. How could I expect someone to love me when I couldn't? I had discovered something raw and true about my thoughts and beliefs that I had never been consciously aware of. That was the beginning of my journey of self-love. The first step is to acknowledge the truth.

I know many people who are living with the belief that they are not good enough or worthy of love. If you are one of them, I want to reach out and hug you because I suspect that you also believed the lies you were told while growing up. Enough is enough- STOP believing the LIES. Decide to start loving yourself as a perfect child of the Universe, of God, of the Divine Source. It doesn't matter if you are a religious or spiritual person or not. It's not about your race, the color of your skin, your ethnic background, your finances or your sexual orientation.

All you need to believe is that you have the power to be joyful and happy. We were created to be resourceful and successful. Our mission-our purpose on this planet-is to learn, grow, and evolve. To be better every day and do the best we can.

Stop judging yourself and start changing the thoughts and beliefs you learned about yourself while growing up. There is a better way to live, dear one. It's time for you to remove the dark and negative glasses you have been wearing and exchange them for a pair that is positive. Wear glasses that enable you to love and adore yourself every single day when you look in the mirror. Because you are truly worthy and deserving of love.

The Uplifting Power of Music and Dance

Another tool I have taught my clients is to listen to uplifting music. I love music; it makes me feel happy, joyful, and alive. It makes me be in the present moment rather than focusing on what I can't change. Depending on my mood, sometimes I listen to relaxing music with the sound of crashing waves on the beach and, other times, I will listen to something more upbeat. It really doesn't matter; it's about you and what makes you happy and present. We need time to be in the moment and forget about life in general. Listen to music that brings you joy rather than the kinds of lyrics that make you think of sad past events.

Speaking of music, I should talk about moving, exercise, and dancing. I love dancing and working out to the sound of happy music. It makes me feel alive no matter what kind of day I had. Sometimes I have to force myself to work out, but once I am done, I feel refreshed and rejuvenated. A healthy mind requires respite. Working out, listening to music, dancing and walking in nature provides more oxygenated blood to move throughout our body and feeds the mind. It allows you to feel vibrant and alive. It also enables you to clear your mind of any negative thoughts and toss aside any negative energy you have experienced in your day.

The Importance of Working with a Coach

I have invested in many coaches for the past twenty years. Truth be told, I have never gone long without working with an expert. It's a necessity for me to be on track and accountable. A trained coach will see your blind spots and assist you to move you out of a slump. I have had coaches for writing, speaking, emotional well-being, exercising, and business. Working with one expert helped me to the next step, ready for the next teacher to come in. I wouldn't be who I am if it weren't for my experienced coaches to get me to the next step.

You may fear that a coach is too expensive. That is really your fear of not being good enough to succeed preventing you from investing in yourself. You spend money in other areas of your life. Are you wasting money on buying coffee when you can make it at home? Are you spending money on unnecessary entertainment? Are you spending money shopping for things you don't need? Do you smoke, drink, or excessively eat out?

Trust me, I am not trying to make your life miserable. I have done all of these in order to survive. I'm not asking you to give up fun but to have fun responsibly – and find the joy or usefulness in even the cutbacks. For example, when I was going to college, I didn't have money to buy a car. I took two buses to go to school and back. I used that time to my advantage to study. It was time-consuming to spend a few hours a day taking buses, but my time was never wasted. I wisely spent it to get me to the next level of success.

I didn't have money to eat out, so my lunch at school was peanut butter and jelly for two years. I am not joking at all. And by the way, I still like peanut butter and jelly!

I used to make sandwiches and take water to the school playground with my children. I would study while they were playing nearby. Almost thirty years later, my children have great memories of playing outside with their friends.

The best mindset coaches are those who are trained in hypnotherapy and have an NLP degree, (they are a neurolinguistic practitioner). I had the opportunity to change my mindset and release many traumas by working with a hypnotherapist for a long time. Some may think of hypnotherapy as stage hypnosis that makes people quack like a duck. Those are just for entertainment. The coaches who are certified in hypnotherapy will help change a client's mindset by having the client relax as they promote positive statements to delve deep within the psyche. You don't need to do anything but simply relax and enjoy the ride.

Keep in mind that hypnosis is not a magic wand. (Yes, I meant it when I said you have to use your tools regularly in order to hold on to that positive mindset!) If someone is not willing to let go of a certain habit, no matter how many sessions they have, they will go back to continue with their habits and old lifestyle. The only time hypnosis works is when someone truly wants to change, consciously desires a better outcome, and puts in the efforts to do so.

There are many more tools and ways to change the mindset to be able to successfully move forward in life. But please remember that it's constant work to acknowledge and understand your mindset. There is no magic remedy to make us feel like superheroes and become successful overnight. There are many aspects of the psyche that affect how we act and react everyday in various situations. As we solve one problem, one more challenge may appear to help us grow and evolve.

Redirecting the Mind

As I have mentioned before in this book, all of the negative chatters in your mind are due to limited beliefs and mindset. Observe them, interpret their meanings, and move from there by taking action every day. If your thoughts are about life-and-death situations, move from the danger. If they are just another way for you to believe you are not good enough, redirect your mind by saying, "Thanks for sharing. I know what I want. I will be fine." Consider your mind and what it's trying to convey to you as a friend who is trying to communicate with you. It may feel strange at first, but you have got to find a common ground with your fears and what your mind is trying to achieve.

That's how I redirect my mind every day. I acknowledge the feelings, and I try to find the meanings. From that place, I know I need to redirect my mind, take action, and move forward to the next step.

Believe in your self-worth. Stop judging and criticizing yourself by believing you are not good enough. Stop making excuses that you are too old, too short, too tall, too big, too small. Be mindful and watch your words, thoughts, and beliefs. Stop shame and guilt; they are components of your past experiences. You are worthy, lovable, good enough, and significant.

Do you have questions or need help regarding your mindset? Send me an email: info@soodabehmokry.com

Are you ready to reach your highest potential, but don't know where to begin? Check my website: www.soodabehmokry.com

You can also connect with me in my FB group: https://www.facebook.com/groups/globalholistichealing/

Chapter Six

Step Four: Awakening the Power of Intuition

It was over thirty years ago, after I graduated from the nursing program in Iran. With war raging, the government had created an intense one-year nursing program to get more of us in the field quicker. I'd gone from that to working the night shift in a university hospital.

Along with two other nurses, I was caring for over thirty patients. There was no doctor present at nights but they were available on call for urgent situations. Our job was to ensure our patients were cared for and ready for procedures or surgery the next day.

I recall events when we asked for the on-call doctor to visit during an urgent situation. I watched the doctors scratching their heads and trying to figure out what was wrong with my patients. Their response seemed strange and frustrating. I was baffled that the doctors didn't know what to do. I would wonder why a doctor who had spent many years in education and training didn't know what to do.

To me, a 20- year-old nurse with only a one-year nursing education, the answer seemed simple. I knew what was wrong with my patient, which organ was affected, and what tests needed to be done. How was I able to know what to do? I had all the answers, and the doctor did not.

"Doesn't it look like the liver maybe is involved?" I would ask the doctor politely, suggesting certain tests to help the patient.

I thought my ability to understand my patient's health was due to the strength of my nursing program and the in-depth way we worked with patients. This was the only conclusion I could reach. I didn't understand that medicine is a head-scratcher, and finding answers takes time and a lot of tests. I was unaware that sometimes even the best doctors won't know the answers.

I questioned the doctor's expertise, and thought they weren't competent enough. I had no idea my knowledge was because of my intuition. I didn't know anything medically either, relatively speaking. My grasp of the situation did not come from physical awareness based in science. I was able to save lives many times by calling the doctor at the right time and discussing what the patient needed because I intuited the problems and solutions. Many years later, I realized I had the honor of being respected by my colleagues, managers, and doctors because of my ability to intervene at the right time. They were exceptional not only for their medical skill but because they listened and accepted what I knew.

I also later discovered that most health care workers are drawn to serve based at least in part on their intuitive guidance. Those who are great at their jobs, are more connected with their intuition, even though they may not be aware of it. Being aware of the power of intuition could save us a lot of headaches and heartaches in life.

My intuition was the only tool I had when I didn't have enough trust or faith in my ability to be and do certain things in life. My intuition gave me a high degree of certainty about what I was being guided to do or say. I couldn't argue or discount those feelings no matter what. They didn't feel like simple thoughts or empty impulses. They felt like a force within me pushing me strongly to act or react suddenly. I would persist until I achieved results.

My intuitive guidance was the reason I felt compelled to make a courageous and bold decision to meet with the director of an American nursing program many years ago. After moving to the States from Iran, I was told I'd have to wait a year before even being eligible to apply to the nursing program. Then the idea to make an appointment with the director of the nursing program popped in my mind one day. I never thought it was a bold decision. It felt natural and necessary to act in this way. I didn't question the idea for even a minute, even as I entered the reception area.

"I would like to make an appointment to talk with the director please." I simply told the receptionist.

"Oh, she is available now. Would you like to see her?"

I was surprised as I accepted the invitation without any hesitation. I met with Maureen, as she introduced herself, who dressed in a black pantsuit, her brown wavy hair pulled back in a ponytail, and her friendly smile put me at ease.

"I am sorry for your experiences so far," she said after I told her my story, "and I'm proud of your accomplishments. To tell you the truth, you are bold, thinking you can enter the program. You haven't completed your pre-requisite classes yet."

"I know. I am well aware of the situation, but I don't have time. I have two young children to take care of and have no time or money to waste waiting to enter the nursing program next year. Please give me a chance, I can prove I was worth the risk."

I had no idea where these words came from. Sitting right here and writing about it, I still have no idea how I decided to take the risk and try to convince Maureen. Except for this: the only explanation is that I followed the guidance of my intuition. It is stronger than my physical ability to negate the feelings.

"Are you going to take other classes in addition to the nursing program? Maureen asked surprised, leaning toward me in her leather chair wondering how I even considered the thought.

"I promise I will make it. I am not afraid of hard work, and I will do whatever it takes. I just can't wait. Please don't make me wait."

Leaning back in her chair, Maureen looked at my transcript and then looked back up at me. "There is a bridge program for licensed practical nurses during the summer. This can prepare you for the second year of nursing school. You could do that."

"Yes, I will do whatever you ask me to."

Her eyes lit up. "I have never met anyone like you, Soodabeh. I am sure you will be very successful." She shook my hand and walked me out the door.

Following the guidance of my soul helped me to get the result I wanted. I decided to start taking the last term of the first-year of the program in spring instead of waiting until summer. Maureen had trusted me. I wanted to show her I was grateful for her kindness and generosity and to prove to her that I was a hardworking person. And I did. The following year, I was able to graduate as a registered nurse!

What's intuition and why is it important?

We are born with innate power and wisdom to guide us through life. Intuition is a natural, normal, and essential part of us. It's our inner guidance system, our instinct, and an indicator trying to communicate what is true beyond what the mind understands. Intuition is essential to successful navigation and creation in our life.

Intuition is our internal GPS; it guides us to where we need to be in life, which direction to go, and which path to take. Life becomes easier and effortless when we awaken our intuition. It allows us to be free by removing all obstacles in our life. We are able to get rid of the clutter and the negative experiences of the past. Being aware of intuition allows us to become one with our spirit and one with the universe, God, higher consciousness, and the Divine Source. We become the powerful spirit shining with more light, life, and brighter than ever before.

We have all experienced intuition at some point in our life. It's when we start thinking of a friend and the phone rings: that friend is calling to say hello. Or, how many times you have known the truth about someone, and you neglected to accept it until it was too late? How many times have you sensed something, good or bad, was about to happen, though you had no idea what or when?

My daughter has always been deeply aware of her intuition, since she was a young child. She was always quite connected to the power and the wisdom bestowed upon us the day we were born.

As a teenager, she would join her brother in laughing and teasing me every time I reminded her that she knew something before it happened because of her intuition. I never felt disrespected though because I knew she would come around. Indeed, now, there is no more laughing about the concept of intuition in my family.

The following story is a perfect example of how our intuition can serve us if we listen to it:

Many years ago I was working the night shift in a hospital . For a week, every time I tried to say goodbye to my daughter before going to work, she would beg me not to go. She had a hunch I would get in a car accident, but she had no idea when.

A few weeks passed, and my daughter and I were leaving my friend's home when we got in a car accident. Everyone who saw the accident believed it was a miracle both of us survived since my brand-new car was completely totaled. My daughter had been sitting in the front passenger seat. I had an intuitive urge to pull her toward me only a minute before the car hit us on the passenger side. My daughter walked away from the accident with only minor scratches on her chest and neck from the seat belt. I shudder to think what would have happened had she been sitting closer to the passenger door at the time of impact.

Discovering the power of intuition grants you the ability to tap into the creative and dynamic self. You will be able to get access to all the knowledge and the wisdom within you. You will begin to feel more powerful when listening to the guidance of your intuition rather than following the fear-based guidance of the confusing mind.

Intuition is about the journey into the core of our being, about self-awareness and honoring who we are. As you acknowledge and follow your intuitive guidance, life becomes full of joy, wonder, and positive experiences.

I didn't know about the power of intuition for many years until after I moved to America. I grew up in a culture where no one talked about intuition, yet my experiences in Iran prepared me to receive messages from my intuition. My experiences there made me very in tune with my inner self. I felt invisible, insignificant, and not good enough growing up. My negative perception about my physical appearance was shaped by everyone telling me I was too short and not pretty. The idea that I wasn't enough was presented to me by others but solidified in my life when I mentally came into agreement with the things that people would say. Once I believed their lies, my mind did a great job at producing thoughts that reinforced my inadequacy.

So, I preferred to be alone and didn't want to socialize with others. Experiencing deep depression after losing my father added to my withdrawal.

Though I can now see the silver lining to these years, I do not wish this situation on anyone. I had no idea how to channel my energies and seek relief. I was constantly thinking about ending my life when I faced any difficulties at home or at school. I felt I didn't belong anywhere. I believed I had no passion or purpose. I had no desire to live an empty life. *Why should I live when no one loves me?*

I had no idea someday these experiences would be the basis of my teaching techniques later in life. Being quiet and not having anyone to talk to or express my feelings to, taught me how to become more intuitive. I learned this without understanding the concept. I would spend time reading and learning from other people's experiences. I loved connecting with nature and walking hours on the beach. It made me feel serene and more connected with the spirit within.

I would watch the branches of a tree and feel the energy and the details of the way the tree was standing still, receiving life force energy from Mother Earth. I remember one day I was sitting in my aunt's back yard. I was so quietly lost deep within my thoughts that I felt the apple tree. I had no idea I was in a meditative state that had allowed me to connect with the essence of the tree. It felt as though the tree were telling me a story, as though I were listening to a friend whispering in my ears.

I now understand that I was being aware of my intuition. Every living and breathing thing is made of energy. We are able to connect with these vast energies every day. That's why nature makes us feel happy and alive. We feel the energies of our plants without being able to explain the phenomenon of how these connections take place.

Intuition in Medical Practice

I remember many years ago when I was working in a skilled nursing facility as a charge nurse. I was working with a doctor who never agreed with what I had to say. (Yes, despite the many open-minded doctors I have worked with, there were some who would never listen!) I intuitively was aware when something was wrong with my patient, but I was often unable to explain it in phone consultations with Dr. Smith based on the science of medicine. It was difficult to convince Dr. Smith based on the information originated from my intuition. I would argue with him to the point it made my manager concerned.

"Soodabeh, stop fighting with the man. You are going to lose your job if you continue fighting with him. He is a doctor, and you are a nurse. Some doctors are not meant to listen to nurses!" Marilyn would tease me, laughing at my persistence.

"Well, that's too bad." I would reply. "You know I am right. He has to accept that nurses are smart too."

Then one day, Dr. Smith and I met. I happened to be the nurse in the nursing station across from the elevator, when the door opened and a six-foot-tall man wearing a dark brown suit stepped onto our floor. "How can I help you?" I said, smiling.

"I am Dr. Smith," he responded. "You must be Soodabeh. I have talked with you several times; now I have a face to refer to when you call," he replied, also smiling.

At first, I wasn't sure what the outcome of the visit would be, but as we reviewed several patients' conditions and how we were caring for them, I felt Dr. Smith became more open to accepting me as his peer rather than his opponent.

"Soodabeh, you seem very knowledgeable," he said. "I appreciate working with you!"

I was blown away to hear him say that. Finally, after a few challenging months, he realized my goal was to help my patients and not to disagree with him. It was the beginning of an amazing journey of working as a team to serve our patients. I would follow my instincts, and the doctor would test and diagnose, often based on information from my gut feeling.

I remember, my mother used to tell me I was stubborn. It was one of my flaws, according to her. However, the day I met Dr. Smith, I realized that being stubborn can be a good thing. If being stubborn means not giving up easily and continuing on until I see a positive result, then I am honored to have that trait. My persistence made me succeed and perform my job the best I could. It was then that I discovered that sometimes our so-called weaknesses (according to others), are the best gifts we could have in life.

Trusting Intuition Could Save Lives

I have always been an avid advocate for my patients. Working as a home health nurse and taking care of patients in their home without a doctor present has been challenging. Sometimes I have to go above and beyond to convince the doctors to intervene and save lives.

I was working with a patient who was battling cancer. Josh had been in and out of the hospital for a few years. He was weak and exhausted.

"Soodabeh, you need to bring your magic wand and help me. I am never going back to that place," Josh told me the first day I met him after he returned from the hospital.

"Josh, I will do my best to keep you out of the hospital. That's the purpose of having care in a home health setting. It's our goal to keep you safe and as independent as possible at home and with your family."

I had been taking care of Josh for a month and he had learned to trust my skills and expertise, even though I had told him I could never promise him a magic wand. He had the most beautiful and supportive family who loved and adored him very much. One day, I got a frantic call from his wife, Kathy. "Soodabeh, Josh's left arm is red from the wrist up to his elbow, but he doesn't want to go to see his doctor. I don't know what to do."

I asked to talk to Josh over the phone. "Listen, Josh. I know you don't want to go to the emergency room because you are afraid that they might admit you back in the hospital again. But you need to go there this time."

"No, Soodabeh. You can't make me go back there. I am tired and just

want to rest," he responded firmly over the phone.

"Josh, you do trust me, don't you? Please listen to what I am going to tell you. There is a possibility you have a blood clot in your arm. Do you know the danger of having a blood clot? The clot can travel into your bloodstream, go directly to your heart, and create a heart attack. It can also travel to your brain and cause a stroke. Is that what you want?"

"Are they going to keep me in the hospital? I am not going to stay there, Soodabeh."

"Josh, please go there and have them test you and see if it's a blood clot first. They can always give you medicine and send you home knowing you have a home health nurse. If they try to keep you there, tell them no, because you have a nurse taking care of you at home. Please believe me when I say you must go now!"

Josh agreed to listen to me since he knew I wouldn't put his life in danger. He knew I had helped him and his family since he was discharged from the hospital. That evening, Kathy called to thank me for convincing him to go.

"Soodabeh, you were right. He did have a blood clot. They said he was lucky to come when he did. It could have killed him!"

I still have the copy of Kathy's email to my manager about the way I cared for Josh.

Every time I hear stories similar to Josh's, I become more and more confident in my ability to intervene and save lives. We are human and face challenges in our daily life while trying to work and take care of others. Not being aware of our intuition and the guidance it gives us, will harm us in the long run. Learning and following the guidance of the wisdom within makes us happier and more joyful even in the face of challenges. Learning to trust that guidance unlocks solutions to the problems we face.

Being in touch with my intuition to help my patients has been rewarding. I am lucky that many health care workers listen to my advice. However, I become deeply anguished knowing they could also use their intuition yet often choose not to. No matter who we are or what we do, there is wisdom to help us prevent difficult situations and avoid harm.

I firmly believe that the primary reason why healthcare providers make deadly mistakes is because they are practicing medicine based solely on science without also giving regard to their intuitive hunches. Health Care practitioners are often exhausted from working long hours. It is very difficult to focus and feel the wisdom of the intuition when working long hours and without proper self-care.

How to Know and Work with Your Intuition

Learning to connect with your intuition allows the spirit within to lead you to where you want or need to be in your life. You learn to be aware of your body, feelings, thoughts, and energy, which ultimately creates freedom and peace in your life. You learn to tune in, trust your instincts, and follow your internal voice. The journey of self-discovery leads to self-empowerment. You become aware of your subtle, internal influences and urges. Your intuition guides and compels you to take certain actions but it's up to you to act on it.

You can use the same tools you learned about mindset in chapter five to gain clarity about the power of the intuition. The same methods of early morning connection and meditation, focusing on gratitude, and journaling can be applied. Doing these things will allow you to master your thought patterns and become connected with the wisdom within.

Your intuition guides you in a repetitive and positive manner. It's always the same message. You won't feel good one day about a situation and different the next day. Feeling different and inconsistent emotions are the direct product of your mind. The intuition guides with the same degree of gentleness and firmness, helping you to discover your answers. Your mind focuses on the fears most of the time.

We know the truth the majority of the time, but we neglect to accept the truth. One way to make sure you believe in your ability to discover and follow your intuition is to start writing. I have always emphasized the importance of writing to gain more clarity. I advise my clients to read their journal once a week. That reinforces the accuracy of their thoughts about a certain subject and establishes trust in our ability to receive guidance.

Start journaling about your thoughts and feelings regarding the events that happen in your day. Have a small notebook and a pen handy at all times and write when an idea comes to mind. Don't judge the thoughts, and don't begin analyzing them, but listen and capture them as they are. You can analyze them when you are going back and reviewing your journal. Trust me, as you discover the accuracy of your thoughts you captured in your journal, you learn to trust your ability to follow the guidance of your intuition.

As you practice being mindful and connected with your inner guidance, you will feel more in touch with who you are. One way to recognize if your feelings and hunches are intuitive or not, is by paying attention to your body and how you feel. Pay attention to all your senses as if you are scanning your body from head to toe. Focus on your thoughts and your belief system. Are they guiding you in a positive manner? Are you feeling at peace with your thoughts?

When you are feeling anxious every time you think about something or someone, it could be your intuition trying to warn you. You might not know the reason, but every time you think about the subject, you feel uncomfortable. Listening to your body is one of the most important keys in discovering about your intuitive guidance.

I love to write about my thoughts and feelings. Writing allows me to find solutions when I am not sure which direction to move towards. I begin by writing the pros and cons of any situation and try to see how I feel about what I have written. Looking at my options while focusing on how every word makes me feel, allows me to gradually find my way.

I have noticed that, when I am too invested in the outcome of a situation, I don't always feel the answer right away. I don't dwell on this because I know the more I persist in connecting with my spirit to find the answer, the more I block the way for my intuition to intervene. I leave the subject for a while and go about my day. I go to the gym, go to work, and allow the answer to come to me naturally rather than forcefully. I have discovered the answer by watching TV sometimes, flipping through magazines or even catching a glimpse of an image of significance. As I have mentioned, the possibilities are endless.

Stop insisting on knowing the answer right away; it doesn't work that way most of the time. Writing opens our mind to receive answers, but we need to be relaxed to notice the answers.

Persistence Pays Off

A long time ago, when I was attending nursing school, one of my advisors taught us to never accept 'no' for an answer. Although our mind is trying to keep us small, our intuition drives us to jump and take a leap of faith when we have to. Our intuition guides us to approach someone and ask for guidance. Trust the guidance and keep moving forward until you get what you want.

Since then, every time a feeling or thought comes to the surface, guiding me to do something, I take a leap and do it no matter how difficult the task. I used to scare my family because, to them, I appeared to be impulsive rather than intuitive. However, after many years of my falling and getting back up again, they learned to accept and trust me to find my way in life. Even though they may have been concerned about my way of life, they knew the outcome would be pure victory in the end.

Be fearless and bold. Be fierce and take actions to achieve all your goals and desires. There may be times you don't get the results you want right away but, as you try more and in spite of any detours, you will get to where you are meant to be. Learn to follow the guidance of your intuition. It will take you to places you never thought were possible!

Chapter Seven

Step Five: Let Go of the Past

The next step to creating a happy and fulfilled life is to let go of what doesn't serve you. Begin by clearing your physical environment and getting rid of the clutter. We tend to collect things over the years and never give up what we are not using. This accumulation of things clogs the energy fields and prevents the flow of positive energy into our life.

I remember when I was in nursing school and raising two young children. I always had difficulty focusing on my homework. I had to clean up my home before I could concentrate. At the time, I thought maybe I was procrastinating doing what I needed to focus on, but I also noticed that I felt more energetic after cleaning and was able to relax with focus and clarity to absorb what I was reading.

I learned years later that I was being affected by the energy of the clutter and intuitively being guided to clean up, so I could concentrate on what was important to me.

This happens because everything is made of energy. Unfortunately, we have turned away from the simplicity of life to accumulate more stuff. But what we are actually doing is adding things that prevent the flow of energy and creativity.

Past experiences also have energy. I had no idea I kept so much negativity inside until one day when I was about to explode. I found myself in my doctor's office to let her know I was significantly depressed to the point I was thinking of ending my life again.

I had everything I had ever wished for. I had accomplished so much in my life: graduated from nursing school, had a job and a brand new car, and was the owner of a beautiful home, but I was miserable. My children were in their teens and didn't need me any longer. I had collected so much *stuff* to prove to myself I was successful, but I was empty inside. None of those things could save my life.

I wrote more in detail about the day I realized why I was so upset in my first book, *Angel Nightingale.* Soon with the help of an amazing coach, books, and workshops, I learned that I needed to start saying goodbye to the past. I realized I didn't have time to grieve for what I had lost: the loss of my father, my brother, the horrific past traumas of war and being tortured, and the loss of my marriage. My spirit was screaming for peace and tranquility, but it was impossible unless I let go of the past. I had been trying to fill the void inside by collecting and buying things I didn't really need.

I began working my way through my garage and closets, this time not with schoolwork as the reason but with cleaning itself as the reason. I found so many magazines I'd never read again (or for the first time), shoes that were in disrepair, and my children's toys that they no longer needed . The clothes I had brought with me from Iran.

Those reminding me of the family and friends I had left behind. I hadn't had time to grieve for those lost relationships because I had to raise my children, learn another language, go back to school, and create a new life and identity. So now, as I cleaned, I was consumed by unwanted emotions, from sadness to anger. There were times I would quit cleaning and start eating to stop the emotions from flowing. Then I would sit there and bawl.

Sometimes I felt numb. I was letting go of what I'd known, but I didn't know who I was anymore. All I knew was that I wasn't the same person I had been many years ago.

Eventually, I found peace in this action. Every time I would decide to clean one room or space in my home, I would say thanks to the things and memories there that got me through the difficult times before letting them go consciously.

I would buy flowers, use essential oils, burn sage, or light candles to bring more light and delicious fragrance to change and uplift my mood.

I am asking you to also do the same. It's not about being obsessed with cleanliness, or focusing all your energy on this subject. But simply the fact that clearing your home's energy allows your creative energies to surface. It is an invitation for positive energy to enter your space, mind, heart, and spirit. If you haven't tried it yet, just experiment and see how it makes you feel. You don't need to take my word for it.

The Importance of Forgiveness

When we hold onto past events and experiences, we can harbor a lot of anger and resentment. Holding onto past trauma is one of the major causes of health issues; physically, mentally, emotionally, and spiritually.

I have worked with clients who consciously or subconsciously are holding on to what they have experienced instead of letting go of the past. They resist letting go of the past because doing so would require that they do something about their present situations.

Holding onto negative experiences gives them purpose and reasons to why they have failed or why they can't move forward. Even though they are hurting and miserable by holding tightly to the memory of the past, they are not willing to forgive and let go.

I remember one of my teachers telling me that I wouldn't be able to help some clients because they are not willing to change. Because subconsciously, there is a reason, an outcome, or a seemingly positive payoff that makes them want to hang on to the past tightly.

Forgiveness is not about forgiving the actions but about letting go of the pain and the heaviness of carrying unnecessary, old baggage. Sometimes it can be hard to use the word *forgiveness*. What has helped me is to say, "I am willing to let go," rather than saying, "I forgive."

I remember, a long time ago, I was struggling to let go of what my ex-husband did. I had moved on with my life, but I was still feeling like I was a victim, recalling what he had done years earlier.

I learned about the book – *Sacred Contract* – by Caroline Myss. This book truly changed my life and the way I viewed past experiences. I realized that what my ex-husband did was a blessing and a gift. He gave me an opportunity to discover my true self, tap into my strength, and learn self-love. I was blessed to start a new life- a new beginning.

I was touched to the point that I decided to write him a letter and let him know I had forgiven him for what he had done. I was ready to let the past go. It wasn't necessary for me to carry it any longer. I decided that I wasn't a victim anymore, but a powerful woman who overcame adversity and created the best life she deserved. That was the beginning of a life filled with freedom and new opportunities for me.

In my private practice working with my clients, I always focus on tools to help my clients to clear their past traumas and negative life experiences. When we hold on to the pain, we prevent positive experiences from entering our life. We can't focus on pain, anger, resentment, and negativity, and expect happiness and love.

What we focus on, we create. Focusing on gratitude creates more positive experiences to be grateful for. Focusing on negative experiences, attracts more negativity into our reality.

To create a healthy and loving experience, you need to let go of what is not working. You can't hold on to grudges, thoughts of blame, and what is wrong in your life, and expect the good experiences to arrive. You must let go of the clutters in your life to allow more positive energy to come in. Working on your mindset allows you to be aware of your self-worth; it allows you to make better choices in life.

Are you having difficulty letting go of the past? I have a special program with proven technique and meditation that has helped many of my clients to clear and heal the negative energy of the past experiences and propel them to live a life filled with freedom, healing, and love.

Are you ready to let go of the past and open your heart fully?

I am here to help and guide you when you decide.

Protect Your Energy Field

We must be aware of negative energy not just from people and things but from information. One of the first things I learned from reading many books on my journey of personal growth was to stop watching or listening to news. The negative energy being broadcasted via the News stations affects what we think and feel about ourselves, the environment, and the world in general. This energy makes us feel uncertain, fearful, stressed, and anxious. When we are focused on negative feelings and energies, we can't enjoy life. This is because we can't focus on fear and pleasure at the same time. When we are afraid due to what we hear or see in the news, we focus on fears, which in turn prevents us from focusing on joy, peace, or happiness.

I noticed that watching the news had increased my susceptibility to additional health issues. Most of the world news focused on criminal activities and acts of violence. Watching and hearing these negative broadcasts made my subconscious mind recall the energy of my own past traumas, which caused me to experience depression and anxiety.

Everything we hear or see affects our brain. The negative energies make us suspicious of people's motives and causes distrust. When we are watching a video, TV, or a movie, we are in a hypnotic state in which the subconscious mind accepts everything it's told. That's how advertising works; it makes us believe we need something when we really don't.

We are constantly focused in two states of being every day. We are either focusing on negativity- the primal state, or positivity- the spiritual state. The primal state is defined as stress, worry, anxiety, overwhelm, anger, indecision, uncertainty, criticizing self or others, comparing yourself to others and feeling inadequate or like you're not good enough. Focusing on the positive and spiritual state of being is defined as hope, gratitude, compassion, generosity, joy, calmness, curiosity, courage, love, certainty, inner peace, art, and creativity.

Today, we have more than just radio and TV news to be concerned about due to increased interactions with social media. We are constantly being bombarded by information that is not aligned with our higher self and well-being.

Our mind stores all of the information and that is the reason for increased turmoil in our lives. That's why we have a lot of children, teenagers, and young adults suffering from fears, anxiety, and depression – it's due to interacting with social media. We may not even be aware of why we feel certain emotions.

Observing and absorbing these messages makes us feel stuck in the primal state and far from reaching our highest potential. We feel powerless, filled with resentment and anger about our perceived state of lack. Watching others going on trips, having fun doing certain activities with family, or enjoying a new job or promotion, can cause envy, jealousy, and feelings of inadequacy. People may wish they had more. There is nothing wrong with wanting to have more from life, but feeling pressure to compare our life with the life of others is not a good way to live.

The truth is that we are created to be happy and peaceful. That's the state of being that we need to create for ourselves every day to allow more creativity to appear in our experiences. Staying away from social media and the news will allow us to be aware of what is going on within us. It's a great way to turn off the unnecessary noise of the everyday hustle and bustle and learn to pay attention to our needs and desires.

However, staying away from social media is not always possible. There are those whose jobs depend on their interactions on social media. So, if you are not able to turn off the bombardment of energy, how do you thrive while watching

negative news stories that add to your stress and social media stories that provoke feelings of inadequacy?

Tools to Protect Your Energy Fields

Being a nurse and a compassionate person, I used to feel the energy of my patients very intensely. Consequently, I would feel so exhausted and drained by the end of each workday that I would sleep on my days off just to recharge before going back to work. Sleeping would counteract my body's absorption of the energy of others. Their pain was making me literally sick and my body was desperately trying to resist it by beckoning me to rest .

One of the most important ways to bring balance and harmony to our being is to reduce the influx of negative energies we encounter daily. There are many ways to protect and clear our energy fields. In previous chapters, I discussed the importance of meditation and visualization. I use these techniques every day to make sure I am protected and clear of unwanted energy so I can focus on my patients and clients. Here are more ideas:

Visualize White Light

One of the tools that works for me is visualizing being wrapped by white light energy. The white light symbolizes protection and healing. It allows me to be clear and focused to help others. Sit in a quiet place and take three deep breaths. Inhale for three seconds through your nose, and exhale slowly for the count of four from your mouth.

Every time you inhale, picture a white light coming down from the Source, God, Universe, whatever you believe in. Allow this light, and its healing energy to move through you from the top of your head to the tip of your toes. Try to sit for ten to fifteen minutes and visualize this relaxing light and energy.

When you are done, you can complete your visualization by imagining the light protecting you in a bubble. You can keep focusing on this light before you enter your work area and interact with others. This even works when you are on the phone. The light will protect your energy field whether you are aware of it or not. You can also ask the light to protect your home, your car, your family, and your friends. I practice protection with light for all of my family and friends every morning and night.

Waterfall Visualization

I learned to visualize being under a waterfall on a tropical island. I love nature and the magic of water washing over me. I visualize the water is mixed with sparkles of white and pink light for healing, clearing, and loving energies. You can practice this every time you take a shower; imagine you are being washed and cleared of any negative energy.

Once you are able to imagine this in the shower, try to visualize the waterfall washing over you every time you feel your energy is being depleted. You can practice this throughout the day and before going to bed. Make a ritual of being aware and conscious of your energy fields daily. You are important enough to do this for yourself.

More Little Ideas That Make a Big Difference

You must begin clearing your internal environment (by releasing all your anger, resentments, grief, and emotional clutter) as well as your external environment by simplifying your life (living area and work environment).

Clear your energy fields through meditation, exercise, dancing, listening to uplifting music, or walking in nature. Surround yourself by lots of plants, flowers, meaningful pictures, and the beautiful scents of essential oils in your home and work area.

Let go of negative people, situations, and toxic work environments. Welcome harmonious, peaceful, and tranquil events and situations. Self-care is very important. Get a massage, manicure or pedicure, or whatever makes you feel good about yourself. You deserve the best.

Chapter Eight

Step Seven: The Importance of Health and Well-being

How much is your health worth to you?

Education is particularly important when it's about our health and well-being.

- All insurance companies, including Medicare, are raising their price causing the quality of care to be the last thing they are concerned about.

- The cost of doctor visits, emergency room services, or hospitalization is increasing every year. This has forced many people to use their assets and lose everything they have earned for many years. Some have become homeless as a result.

- The health care practitioners are overwhelmed, stressed, and burned out.

- Mistakes happen because those who care for you are tired, stressed, and overwhelmed by the constant demands of a job that is more focused more on productivity than quality care.

Why do you need to wait until you are sick to finally decide to take care of your health?

You matter. Your physical, emotional, and mental health and well-being is important.

You don't deserve to constantly battle with health issues; waking up with low energy, an inability to focus and feeling unfulfilled.

My personal experience with health issues and working as a nurse for over thirty years has taught me so much. When I was working in the hospital, I would only see patients for a short period of time when they were sick. Then they would be discharged from the hospital and I might never see them again.

Working as a home health nurse for over twenty years has opened my eyes. I learned how people live, what they know about their health, what they eat, and so much more. I learned the majority of these people were left uninformed about their illness in many areas and with little to no understanding of what caused their sickness. This is because no one had the time to talk with them to find the underlying issues that caused them to be sick in the first place. I can't emphasize how many times patients asked me, "Why didn't my doctor tell me this?"

My only response was that they probably didn't have time to discuss it with you.

We have a mindset of believing our doctors know what's wrong with us because we were told that was the case. Trust me, I have nothing against doctors. However, we need to understand that doctors are authorized fifteen minutes to see each patient, discuss the symptoms, and prescribe medications.

How many times have you heard a doctor asking you what you eat every day? How many meals do you eat and what is in each meal? How many doctors have told you the side effects of any medications? It's up to us to get this information in a piece of paper from the pharmacist, right? How many of you are reading the information?

I had patients read the information about their medications and decide they weren't willing to take the medications the doctor prescribed for them because they feared the side effects written on the paper just handed to them. Unfortunately, the doctors don't have time to discuss any of these concerns with their patients.

Stress and Health Issues

Let me first start by saying that I do not diagnose, treat, or cure any health issues. I know the reason why we get sick, however. My goal is to prevent health issues. This is my passion and purpose: to have people be informed. It's time to be responsible and accountable for our health and well-being. We need to take initiative and make informed decisions regarding our life rather than wait until we are sick and at the mercy of someone who doesn't know anything about our life.

Let me tell you a story from my personal experience. I have a form of autoimmune disease which means my body attacks its cells and organs. Sometimes the issue affects my joints, muscles, stomach and so forth. I had a cortisone injection in my knee when I was thirteen years old. I had issues with bleeding from my stomach when I was in my early twenties, and I underwent radiation due to overactive thyroid glands when I was in my early thirties. The list goes on and on...

Working full-time and raising two young children as a single mother was extremely stressful for me. I had no family support to help me with financial stress or to help me with the emotional stress of the constant demands in my life. I used to work long hours and then come home to take care of my children. I was always tired and fatigued every day. My life was draining my energy, and I didn't know how to get better.

I would sleep for hours when I could and when I was off. It was an endless cycle of working non-stop and crashing. I felt defeated and thought I had failed my children. I was not able to be present for my children 100 percent of the time because I didn't have the energy or stamina at the end of the day.

When I was introduced to the concept of how stress affects our health, I thought I had found the solution for my health issues. Growing up, I experienced a lot of traumas which caused my body to exhibit health issues. My body couldn't tolerate any more stress and trauma, so it was manifesting as symptoms of a different illness.

I believe our body is smart. Our body speaks to us constantly. The pain we feel in our body means that we have done something which pushed our body past its limit. When we eat certain food then get an upset stomach, it's our body telling us that that particular food is not good for us. When we are smoking and then begin to cough as a result, it's our body communicating to us that smoking is affecting our lungs.

We have a tendency to ignore these symptoms and continue doing what we are doing until we get sick and need medication to mask the pain and symptoms our body uses to communicate with us. We try to numb the pain and shut the voice within us so we can continue doing what is harmful for our body.

The doctor gives us medications that affect other organs in our body and we keep going until our body and all of the organs shut down completely.

In my job as a home health nurse, I see patients suffering, taking twenty to fifty medications, and still not getting adequate results. I have witnessed many occasions when the only remedy was to discontinue all medications and start all over again. A majority of the time patients felt better when the doctor decided to cut back all or most of their medications. Trust me, I am not against taking medications as needed for our health issues. My goal is to help people to prevent health issues.

What is Stress and How it Affects Us

Stress is a normal and natural physical response. Stress is not always a bad thing and can be seen as useful when we are in basic survival mode. It's a brilliant way to warn us when we are facing potential danger. During a stressful situation, our body activates its fight-or-flight system in order to keep us safe.

This phenomenon results in the release of hormones and chemicals such as adrenaline, cortisol, and norepinephrine so that the body can act and respond quickly in the face of the harmful situation. It causes increased blood flow to muscles, which results in higher heart rate and increased breathing to give us more energy to either fight the danger or run away to save our life.

The Effect of Modern-Day Stress

We all have obligations to our family, friends, and our work. Many people work more than one job to make ends meet. Working too much to provide for our family, meeting deadlines, and dealing with the demands of raising children are the causes of modern-day stress.

We are expected to do more than we are physically able to. Facing these challenges and not having time to take care of ourselves increases the stress level.

Experiencing constant stress for a long time causes the body to act as though it is facing a dangerous situation, which leads to it releasing more hormones and chemicals into the bloodstream. The elevated cortisol level leads to health issues such as heart disease, stroke, diabetes, digestive issues, depression, anxiety, insomnia, chronic pain, auto-immune disease, and even cancer. People respond to stressful situations differently. The effects of stress can manifest as physical, emotional, or behavioral issues. Some people may become agitated and demonstrate aggressive behaviors at home or work, creating unsafe environments and leading to violence. Others may choose addictive behaviors, such as drinking alcohol, eating too much food, shopping, or gambling.

Step Eight: How to Manage Your Stress

Although we may not be able to avoid stress, there are many ways to minimize and manage its effect:

Gratitude

Focus on the present moment and be grateful for what you have. Take a few moments each morning before getting out of bed and at night before going to sleep to focus on positive. Have the intention of creating a peaceful and productive day and a restful sleep. The more you focus on gratitude, the more positive experiences you will attract in your life.

Express Your Emotions

One of the most important ways to deal with stress is to express feelings and emotions in a healthy manner. Living in my birth country with its very strict culture, I had learned to keep everything bottled up. I was told not to tell anyone if I was upset, sick, or even unhappy. My only defense mechanism was to work harder to prove my worth.

Trying to become healthier, I realized that I needed to express my emotions and find a healthy way to let go of the past. I had stuffed down many years of pain, which had manifested as physical pain all over my body.

Journaling helped me to express my feelings. Once I was able to express and release my feelings, I felt better and lighter.

Create Healthy Boundaries.

It's very important to have healthy boundaries. People are not mind readers. If you don't have any boundaries, you will be tired and stressed. It is important to say yes to yourself, taking time to relax and rejuvenate. Saying no to what you can't do or don't want to do is a great way of creating healthy boundaries. You are the only one who knows what you can or can't do. Taking care of yourself is a must and a key to managing your stress level.

Take Time to Play

I didn't like a lot of physical exercises growing up, but I loved to dance. I was able to express myself in a way that was safe for me. Dancing was my way of playing. Even to this day, every time I dance, I feel like a child.

Spending time and playing with my granddaughters makes me feel absolutely joyful. It warms my heart to see them happy and healthy; to experience pure, unconditional love is bliss. No matter what play means to you, find a way to do so. Whether playing with your children, grandchildren, or even pets, just do it.

Participate in Physical Activity and Exercise

I was elated to discover Jazzercise. It wasn't exercise to me, but music and dancing. Before Jazzercise, I used to walk a lot. I have loved walking since I was a young girl, especially walking on the beach. Walking helped me to calm down, find creative solutions, and connect with my spirit. No matter what form of exercise you choose, make sure it's something you like and enjoy. Exercise releases chemicals called endorphins, which results in triggering positive feelings in the body. The endorphins also interact with the brain receptors to reduce pain.

Connect with Nature

I love outdoor activities. Whether it's walking on the beach, hiking, or gardening, I am always happy when I connect with Mother Nature. Being outside helps me to feel grounded, energized, and reconnected with the powerful spirit within.

Listening to Music

Listening to positive and uplifting music has always made me feel good. Regardless of the genre, so long as it's not stress inducing or filling your mind with negative information, music can be healing. It plays an important key in your well-being.

Guided Imagery and Meditation

I had a difficult time quieting my mind when I tried to meditate. However, when I learned about guided imagery, I discovered the best way to focus my mind. There are many different guided imagery and meditation audios available these days. It really doesn't matter which one you choose – they all will help you to feel serene and peaceful. When we are stressed, we hold our breath. Both meditation and guided imagery focus on breathing exercises, which allow the oxygenated blood to circulate to our internal organs, especially our brain.

Healthful Eating Habits

Preparing healthy food and paying attention to your nutrition are a must. Working as a home health nurse requires that I do a lot of driving so I don't often have a place to sit down and enjoy my meals. However, I have learned to be prepared. I have fruit, vegetables, nuts, and nutrition bars with me to munch on during the day to keep me satiated so I will have more energy. Going without food leads to low blood sugar, which makes the body feel sluggish, so we eat more when we get home. Consuming more sugar and carbohydrates may make us feel good at first due to an increase in blood sugar, but then we crash down a few hours later. This increases the risk of insulin-resistant diabetes, heart issues, stroke, chronic pain, depression, and anxiety.

Contrary to this, eating more leafy vegetables and protein helps to increase energy and stabilize moods.

Complementary and Alternative Medicine

There are many ways to reduce and manage your stress. Massage, acupuncture, comfort touch, Reiki, aromatherapy, and hypnosis are all beneficial for stress management and overall well-being. As a nurse and certified hypnotherapist, I specialize in stress management techniques. For more information, visit my website at www.soodabehmokry.com

Or email me: info@soodabehmokry.com

Chapter Nine

Step Nine: Embracing Change

Change is a constant part of life. It's a natural and vital process for us to grow and evolve. Seasons change, day changes to night, and everything around us is constantly evolving. Sometimes we resist change because of a lack of confidence and a low self-esteem; not believing that we are worthy of having the best life we want and deserve. I never liked change and used to always complain about it. I didn't know it was necessary and crucial sometimes.

I stayed in unhappy relationships for the fear of not being able to find someone better. I tolerated bullies at work because I was scared that I wouldn't find a better job. It took me many years to understand that change was inevitable and often the catalyst to the most wonderful events in my life. I learned to embrace change the hard way!

The Desire to Change

I woke up with a sharp pain in my right hand and couldn't move it in any direction. I was in tears, running to my daughter and asking her to help me to get dressed and take me to the doctor's office.

"What happened," the doctor said.

"I have no idea, I woke up with the pain," I said while in tears.

"what do you do?"

"I am a nurse."

She looked at me and smiled. "I've seen this before. Do you really think it just happened for no reason?"

I had no idea what was going on, I just wanted the pain to stop so I would be able to go back to work the next day. I had no idea it was the beginning of a long journey for me. My life changed from working every day and doing what I really loved to daily trips for physical therapy, occupational therapy, chiropractic, massage, acupuncture, orthopedic and neurological services, and much more.

The pain persisted, radiating to my elbow, upper arm, shoulder, and all the way to my neck. And eventually it was replaced by tingling and numbness. I had to wear a long splint from my upper arm to my fingers. In spite of all the tests, some more painful than others, no one could understand what was wrong with me.

I was depressed and desperate for an answer, crying all the time. I feared being disabled for the rest of my life. I began to pray, mediating every night, asking for guidance. One night during my meditation, I was guided to start writing. I was surprised, and I thought it was my imagination. I heard the voice again, "you need to start writing."

"What is this? Don't you see that I can't do anything with my right hand? How can I write with this splint?" I was irritated.

But the voice didn't leave me, and I knew I had to remove the splint and at least try. It was the beginning of a beautiful journey for me. Every night I would meditate and write messages from the spirit and angelic realm. The messages were inspiring and heartwarming. I would look forward to my nightly meditation and listening to the voice of my angels.

One night, I was sitting and watching TV aimlessly and flipping the pages of a nursing magazine. Most of the time, I would toss them in a recycling bin, but that night was different. I suddenly felt as if I was searching for something specific. And suddenly, I stopped when I saw an ad for the *American Holistic Nurses Association.*

I was shocked. I ran to my computer and started searching. It was what I wanted and needed. It was the answer to my prayers. I signed up instantly, so excited to learn more about this organization. A few weeks later, I received the first publication: *Beginnings.*

I found an article about a company using integrative therapy. It was my dream job. I had been trying to incorporate integrative therapy in my nursing practice, but it wasn't allowed or accepted where I was working at that time. I loved my coworkers and the company I was working with, but the dream of working where I could grow, learn, and be able to help people more was very intriguing. I knew I had to leave. Not only leave the job, but leave to another state to work with the other company.

That was the guidance of my soul. I could feel it with every cell in my body and my being. I had to take a leap of faith. I was frightened and didn't know what to do at first. I kept asking for more signs and more guidance, and finally, I decided to go. (I have included more stories about this specific journey in my first book, *Angel Nightingale.*

I realized if I denied and ignored the guidance of my spirit, I would be forced to face my illness differently. My hand began to completely heal soon after I accepted and embraced my situation. I learned to love and honor myself, to take better care of my needs. I began to devote time to sit still and meditate every night and write the messages of love and inspiration in my journal.

I realized that I had neglected myself for a long time. I didn't take a break and had been working long hours. I loved my job; it didn't seem like "work" to me. But it didn't matter. I needed to take time to reflect on my life, check in and hear the guidance of my intuition, and be ready to follow the voice of the spirit.

The spirit knows what we need, which direction to go, what is needed for our growth and higher self. When we are busy and unable to take a chance to notice, we are forced to face the challenges and obstacles that drive us to seek wisdom from the spirit. I learned to listen and pay attention. I decided to say "No" when I couldn't or didn't want to do something. I learned to honor myself and my spirit. I learned that what didn't kill me made me stronger. I found courage and became empowered to know that I was deserving of having the best in life.

Although it is scary at times, embracing change will open the doors to happiness and success. We are afraid of the unknown and of not being able to see what is out there for us. However, once we decide to accept it, we realize that it is the most wonderful and rewarding event.

Change is a natural process. It means that we are growing, becoming wiser, stronger, and getting closer to finding our mission and purpose in life. Like a butterfly ready to be free. And freedom is the most wonderful thing.

We become consumed when we dwell on the past or future while forgetting to be present and enjoy life. When we focus on being present, we aren't focused on the future to be afraid of the unknown. As we quiet our minds and become still, the answer and guidance will flow naturally and freely. Be still and listen to the wisdom of your soul. The answer is within you. Don't try to force things to happen. Sometimes you can't hear the guidance right away, but it will come to you later. Maybe in your dreams, while watching your favorite TV show, or listening to a song. There are signs everywhere. You'll know when you see it; something within you will notice it and you'll feel it with your heart and soul.

Life would be boring if we knew everything in advance. There would be no fun, surprises, or joy in knowing every little detail of our life. We are the creator of our lives. We have the power to manifest everything we need and want. This is our birthright. It took me many years to finally believe and understand this concept. I know when I don't pay attention, I face the challenge. But I also know that I am able to break free and conquer anything that comes my way when I embrace the situation.

Believe in yourself and the guidance of your spirit. Don't worry. Leave behind the old belief that doesn't serve you. Don't be afraid to take a chance. Be bold, take a risk, and try new things. Don't procrastinate because you are afraid. There are lessons to be learned in order to grow and flourish. Take a leap of faith and follow your bliss. You will see magic unfold right before your eyes. I promise.

Embrace the change!

Chapter Ten

Step Ten: Lead with Love

We are living in a world with hatred, prejudice, discrimination, chaos, and war. Empathy is lacking these days. Families and friends are divided. Everyone is fighting to be right, attacking others with anger, rather than listening to one another with kindness and love.

We have become divided and intolerant of each other. Some began to bully those who have different ideas. Others believe they are superior because of the color of their skin, social status, or money. How did we get here? How can we get to a place of acceptance and empathy for all of our fellow human beings? After all, we are human, with the same anatomy and physiology.

It's hard for me to comprehend what has happened. Because this wasn't my experience twenty-nine years ago when I came to America. I wouldn't have survived without the constant help and support of strangers coming into my life to show me the way. They accepted me for who I was. They opened their heart and their home. They loved me unconditionally and helped me to find my way out of the darkness.

Growing up in Iran and before the revolution took place, I was taught that everyone was the same. My parents were the most loving and generous individuals who taught me to be kind and loving. I remember both my parents always helped those who were unable to provide for their family. We weren't rich. We were a hardworking, middle-class family.

I inherited this love, compassion, and generosity. When my father died, my mother had to work two jobs to meet our family's needs. My father believed strongly in the idea that, when you give much, you receive much. He used to tell my mother that we would never go without.

"Don't worry. We will always have whatever we need. The same way I help others, God will always take care of my family." He was right. Although my mother had to work two jobs, we never went to bed hungry. We always had a roof over our head and clothes on our back. We always had enough. We weren't rich, but we had enough to live like others.

Hopeful and Optimistic

I wonder why people have changed suddenly. Was this hatred in their hearts before but no one was aware of it? How did we get here? How can we establish acceptance and empathy for others as the societal norm? Where do we go from here?

I believe we need to rise up, be the voice of reason, and be the shining light the world needs. We need to unite, to be the ambassadors of love, compassion, and peace. We owe it to our children and grandchildren who have to deal with this chaos. They are our responsibility. They need safety, understanding, and love.

Our nation and the world needs more love, compassion, and empathy. Many are lacking these attributes. What can you do to bring light and love to this world today? Just be positive, be understanding, listen to the voice within you and move forward. Be fearless, be a peaceful warrior.

I vote to reunite based on the love within all of us. The love we are born with; the light in all of us as spirits living in physical form. I am positive and optimistic about our future. Because we are the future. Because I believe *love* is the answer. You can't go wrong with love. Love doesn't see color. Love accepts all. Love doesn't judge. This *love* comes to us from the eternal love of the creator, the Divine Source.

Why is Love the Answer?

Love starts with loving yourself; respecting, and honoring your feelings, your heart, your body. Your self-worth depends on you loving yourself. Be true to yourself. Know you are significant. You matter. Your feelings and emotions matter.

Love is within you, and love is around you. You are a being of love, and you are made of pure love. Divine love resides within you and will never leave you or die. It's up to you to view yourself as perfect the same way the Creator and angels do. It is only when you are not operating in spirit that you can see your imperfections and judge your body based on the lies you were told by society, parents, family, and friends.

You may believe you don't need anyone to help you. You feel asking for help is a sign of weakness. You may even try to protect your heart from getting hurt again.

Maybe you don't believe in your ability to be independent, strong, and powerful. You may feel the need to have someone take care of you because you believe you are unable or not good enough to make decisions about your life.

Either way, these thoughts and beliefs are based on fears and feelings of inadequacy, insignificance and unworthiness. As you change your perspective and begin to incorporate new thoughts and beliefs about yourself, love, and relationships, your experiences change. As you start your new life; the journey of self-discovery, and self-love, you begin attracting experiences that prove you are worthy and deserving of love. Start to view yourself the way your creator and angels see you; beautiful, perfect and worthy to give and receive love.

Focus on who you are, what you want, your dreams and desires. It's not about the look. It's not about the money. It's about what you think of yourself and your worth. You are deserving. You can manifest everything you need and desire. Have healthy boundaries and stop allowing others to take advantage of you. The right person will love you just the way you are.

Allowing people to treat you with respect and dignity should be your number one priority because you are worthy of being treated with love and respect. Be proud of who you are and what you have accomplished. Speak your truth with love and compassion for self and others. Never compromise your morals and values due to the fear of not being liked or loved by anyone. It's not necessary.

You Are Never Alone

God, Divine Source, spirit, and angels are always guiding and directing us. We are surrounded by angels and guides that are ready to help and support us in our journey. It doesn't matter who you are, what color your skin is, what you believe, where you came from. Your angels and guides never leave your side.

Angels don't have feelings or emotions as humans do. There is nothing that could disappoint them, even when you don't follow their guidance. They always see you as a perfect being. However, we are created with the gift of free will. That means no one, not even angels could intervene if we don't ask for help. It's up to us to decide if we want to hear and follow their guidance.

Do you believe in angels? Do you want to learn more? I have inspiring and heart-warming stories of healing with angels in my first book, *Angel Nightingale.*

I share my story to let you know that I feel your pain. I have felt discouraged, frustrated and hopeless. That is why I am so grateful that I allowed the divine to lead me to the answers. I want you to believe you are never alone. Not only do you have divine guidance waiting to show you your next step in life, I am also here for you if you need anything.

I experienced pain, loneliness, loss, and depression. I was told I wasn't good enough, smart enough or strong enough. I was told I couldn't make decisions and wouldn't be able to make it alone. I was laughed at when I shared that I was going back to school in a new country. I was mocked for not being able to speak English. I was told I would fail.

I felt powerless, lost, and confused. I was overwhelmed with all the challenges and struggles I had to face. I felt lonely, isolated, and alone. I had no reason to live.

Somehow deep within, I knew there was a better way to live. I refused to believe I was destined to fail. The more they bullied me, the stronger I became. I realized it was time to change my thoughts and beliefs. Searching for answers led me to learn about the angelic realm. That was the beginning of a magnificent life. I was able to say goodbye to my painful past experiences to replace the pain and anger with love and forgiveness.

Life is complicated and messy sometimes. It is definitely not a fairytale. Overcoming life challenges I discovered there is no failure, but learning lessons. Sometimes we may detour, but with the right mindset, dedication, determination, and perseverance, we learn to succeed and achieve our goals. I learned I am the creator of my own life and powerful enough to manifest everything I desire and more.

It took me many years to finally find myself, my passion, and life purpose. I feel alive and fulfilled living life the way I was meant to live. I love who I have become as a result of my challenges and struggles. I know I am not a victim of my circumstances nor am I just a survivor- I am a victor.

I take my job seriously. I take human life seriously no matter the color of their skin, their sexual orientation, religious beliefs, or ethnicity. I am loving, kind, and generous. I have been working every day to be a better person. I desire to be the one who promotes peace, empathy and kindness. I am the messenger of love and peace. I believe LOVE is the answer, now and forever.

Conclusion

Life is not always easy or fair. We face challenges and roadblocks; we struggle sometimes trying to make sense of what is going on in our life. In the midst of all these changes, you must remember that you are still in control. Even though it may seem the opposite, even though you may feel defeated and hopeless. Even though it may feel like you have lost everything and are alone without any support. The 'happily ever after' that you worked so hard for suddenly was replaced by a nightmare, something you never thought possible.

But you can make a decision; you are free to choose something different, or even better. It may not be easy, but it's possible.

We tend to stay where we feel comfortable even if it is different and painful because it is familiar. Although experiencing life-changing events is painful, difficult, and overwhelming, there is always a solution and a better way to live. Change is often a blessing in disguise.

There is nothing more important than you. If you are not happy or healthy, you won't be able to take care of your family or loved ones. When I was at my lowest point after Hameed told me that he was leaving me, I was helped when I remembered that my children were the most important people in my life. They were the only family I had in America. They were the main reason I was living, breathing, and alive. I was responsible for their happiness and well-being.

I had to change and be accountable for the life I had created for them. It was not my fault their father decided to leave, but it would have been my fault to stay in that toxic relationship blindly hoping for a change, believing he would come back to his senses. I could have stayed in that marriage for years, living with Hameed as roommates and never questioning the emotional and physical distance between us. But that wasn't what I wanted so I searched for answers. Once I was faced with the truth, I had to take the first step to at least accept that my marriage was over.

No matter what your situation is, the first and the most important step is to acknowledge and accept your situation. Don't walk with a blindfold on, hoping something different will happen, or falsely wishing someone will rescue you. Unless you accept and let go of the unhealthy situation, you won't be able to move forward and succeed. You will be wasting time and energy focusing on what will never serve you. You will be depressed; living in fear, anxiety, and depression. And most of all, you will get older regretting the decisions you made based on fears.

I have met many people living in rage, anger, and resentment for years because their partners left them for someone else. I was one of them. It's expected that we will go through the stages of grief no matter what the situation is. However, willingly deciding to stay in grief and refusing to move forward because of something your mother, father, or partner did or said will never serve you in any shape or form.

There is help available. I wasn't just miraculously able to forgive and forget then move on with my life. It was a painful experience losing my father, and my brother, and then, leaving my family, my country, my home, my belongings, and everything I had for a dream. The dream of living a life filled with freedom and peace with my husband and family – which swiftly dissolved into harsh reality. It took me many years to finally be able to move on, to be able to forgive my ex-husband, and to allow myself to enjoy life fully.

For me, holidays were the worst time for many years. I found out on Thanksgiving Day– my first holiday in the States after only a few weeks here – that my husband of ten years was having an affair. Then, I realized my marriage was truly over only a few weeks before celebrating my first Christmas in America. Can you imagine going through holidays year after year remembering how your life changed drastically in a foreign land and, on top of that, being unable to buy any gifts for your children during those gift-giving holidays because that change of circumstances ruined your finances? Can you imagine how my children felt every year not being able to celebrate the holidays with both parents?

It was horrible and dreadful to go through holidays for many years, seeing all the lights and the joy of others looking forward to celebrating the holiday season. I wished I could run away somewhere and hide until the holidays were over. I would cry myself to sleep every single night for many years.

And then, one year, I didn't.

The pain doesn't necessarily go away all at once when you decide to move forward. It will probably linger, but it subsides as you try to get accustomed to your new life. If you allow yourself to grieve and do the work to heal, your new life eventually becomes more joyful than sorrowful. You will smile in acknowledgement of your victories along the way.

I want to let you know that you don't have to suffer anymore. There is a better way for you to live, because you deserve to be happy, healthy, and fulfilled. I am getting older, but I feel I have more energy now than I did when I was in my twenties and thirties. I feel happy and content with my life. Happiness is not about our material worth; it's how we feel inside that matters.

Do you feel good about yourself? Do you feel content with where you are in life? Are you fulfilled? If not, what do you desire? What do you want to change in your life? Do you want to serve more, or do you wish to receive more?

The truth is that all is possible for you, for me, for all of us. We deserve to be happy, healthy, and fulfilled. The first step is to love yourself, believe in yourself, and know that you matter. You were not born to suffer, but to be happy.

Sometimes, we need to look at life with a different perspective. Look at what we have and be grateful for all of it; the good, the bad, and the ugly. Without ALL your life experiences, you wouldn't be who you are. So, embrace it, embrace YOU. Embrace every life event as a beautiful and magnificent gift bestowed upon you by your creator. A gift to shape you into the person that you were meant to be. Say yes to yourself. Say yes to life, your life, the life you have created, and the life you wish to create.

What do you desire? What do you dream of having, experiencing, being, or doing? The time is now. You matter, you are significant, you are important. Start today. One simple step, it's all you need. You deserve it all. I am here to tell you that all is possible for you. The choice is yours. Say yes today.

Speaking of my experience, my intention for sharing it is to let you know that life is not always easy for any of us. It's messy, challenging, dark, and painful – for all of us at certain times. But we survive, we thrive, and we realize the only hero we need is the one who resides within each of us.

Go ahead and decide that your life is going to change today. The past is behind you. There is a new beginning and a dawn awaiting you when you acknowledge and accept what is right at this moment. I am here when you decide. Please remember that you matter, you are resilient, you are significant, and you are deserving of living the life you were created to lead. It's all in your capable hands. The choice is yours. Make a decision today. I will show you the rest. I promise – just believe!

About the Author

Soodabeh Mokry is a Registered Nurse, certified hypnotherapist, experienced holistic wellness coach and passionate speaker. She is also the author of the immigration memoir, *Angel Nightingale*, which inspires her patients and readers to a new level of understanding of the resilience of the human spirit – and inspires them on to action.

Soodabeh is the epitome of an American dream. Her dream of a happy life in the United States as a refugee from Iran was replaced by a nightmare when her marriage ended shortly after she arrived. She was left alone with two young children, no money, no family or friends, and the challenge of learning a new language.

By sharing her personal story of faith, courage, perseverance, and overcoming adversity, Soodabeh inspires people to move beyond our limitations to create lives we desire.

Supported by her thirty years of medical experience and the data behind both Western and alternative wellness techniques, Soodabeh empowers people by providing the step-by-step tools to achieve our goals.

Soodabeh has worked with people suffering with heart disease, diabetes, cancer, depression, anxiety, and chronic pain – many of whom come to her after other attempts and relapses. Soodabeh believes that there is always hope, and she is committed to helping people live healthy and happy lives.

We are each born with the power, passion, and determination to experience a harmonious and fulfilled life. Sometimes our challenges seem to prevent us from reaching our full potential. Limited thoughts and beliefs that we learn from our parents and communities may encourage us to give up and settle for less.

But Soodabeh's message in her patient sessions, presentations and programs, and writing is this: You are not bound by any circumstances. You are capable of manifesting and creating the life you want. You own the power to create your destiny!

About Defining Moments Press

Built for aspiring authors who are looking to share transformative ideas with others throughout the world, Defining Moments Press offers life coaches, healers, business professionals, and other non-fiction or self-help authors a comprehensive solution to get their book published without breaking the bank or taking years.

Defining Moments Press prides itself on bringing readers and authors together to find tools and solutions

As an alternative to self-publishing or signing with a major publishing house - we offer full profits to our authors, low-priced author copies, and simple contract terms.

Most authors get stuck trying to navigate the technical end of publishing. The comprehensive publishing services offered by Defining Moments Press mean that your book will be designed by an experienced graphic artist, available in printed, hard copy format, and coded for all eBook readers, including the Kindle, iPad, Nook, and more.

We handle all of the technical aspects of your book creation so you can spend more time focusing on your business that makes a difference for other people.

Defining Moments Press founder, publisher and #1 bestselling author, Melanie Warner, has over 20 years of experience as a writer, publisher, master life coach and accomplished entrepreneur.

You can learn more about Warner's innovative approach to self-publishing or take advantage of free trainings and education at:MyDefiningMoments.com

Defining Moments Book Publishing

If you're like many authors, you have wanted to write a book for a long time, maybe you have even started a book... but somehow, as hard as you have tried to make your book a priority - other things keep getting in the way.

Some authors have fears about their ability to write or whether or not anyone will value what they write or buy their book. For others, the challenge is making the time to write their book or having accountability to finish it.

It's not just finding the time and confidence to write that is an obstacle. Most authors get overwhelmed with the logistics of finding an editor, finding a support team, hiring an experienced designer, and figuring out all the technicalities of writing, publishing, marketing and launching a book. Others have actually written a book and might have even published it, but did not find a way to make it profitable.

For more information on how to participate in our next Defining Moments Author Training program visit: www.MyDefiningMoments.com. Or you can email melanie@MyDefiningMoments.com

Other Books by Defining Moments Press

- Defining Moments: Coping With the Loss of a Child - by Melanie Warner

- Defining Moments SOS: Stories of Survival - by Melanie Warner and Amber Torres

- Write your Bestselling Book in 8 Weeks or Less and Make a Profit - Even if No One Has Ever Heard of You - by Melanie Warner

- Beyond Brilliant: Roadmap From Fear to Courage – by Shiran Cohen

- Rise, Fight, Love, Repeat: Ignite Your Morning Fire - by Jeff Wickersham

- Life Mapping: Decoding the Blueprint of Your Soul - by Karen Loenser

- Ravens and Rainbows: A Mother-Daughter Story of Grit, Courage and Love After Death – by L. Grey and Vanessa Lynn

- Pivot You! 6 Powerful Steps to Thriving During Uncertain Times – by Suzanne R. Sibilla

- A Workforce Inspired: Tools to Manage Negativity and Support a Toxic-Free Workplace – by Dolores Neira